ATKINS DIET BOOK FOR WOMEN OVER 60

A Low-Carb Guide to
Vibrant Living, Hormonal Harmony, and Sustainable
Wellness for Women Over 60

PEYTON AUDREY

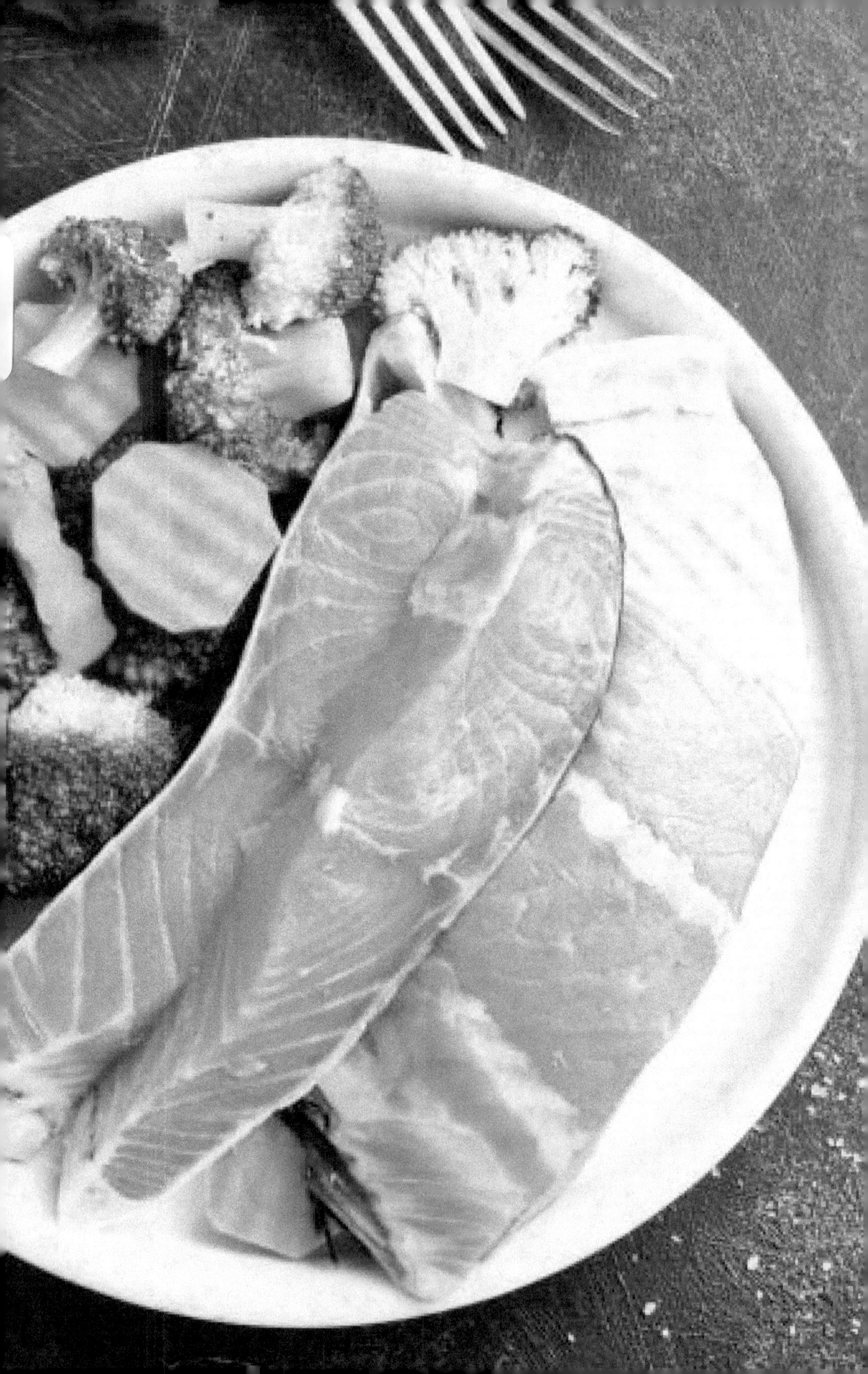

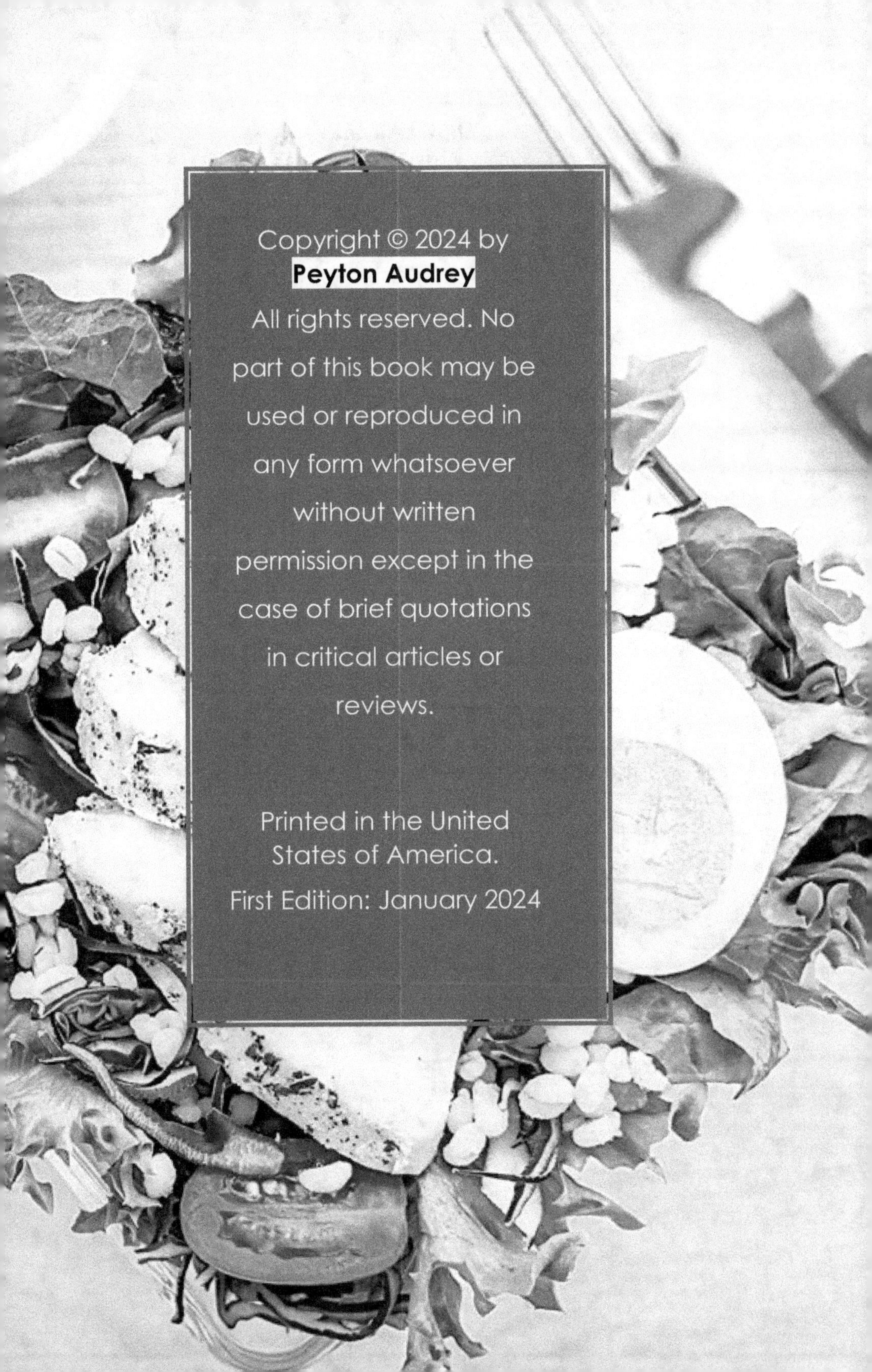

TABLE OF CONTENT

INTRODUCTION

Welcome to the vibrant world of " Atkins Diet Book for Women Over 60: A Low-Carb Guide to Vibrant Living, Hormonal Harmony, and Sustainable Wellness for Women Over 60"! As we gracefully navigate the tapestry of life, it's essential to embrace each chapter with vitality, wisdom, and a dash of rebellious spirit. This book is your passport to a healthier, more vibrant life tailored explicitly for the fabulous women in their golden years.

In the bustling realm of health and wellness, one size doesn't fit all, especially when it comes to the unique needs of women over 60. We understand the challenges you face – from metabolic mysteries to the intricate dance of hormones, bone health concerns to the ever-elusive quest for sustained energy. That's why this isn't just another diet book; it's your personalized guide to rewriting the script on aging.

Embark with us on a journey that transcends mere weight loss. It's about reclaiming your power, embracing the changes, and living life to the fullest. We delve into the science-backed strategies of the Atkins Diet, reshaping them to cater specifically to the incredible women who've seen it all, done it all, and are ready for the next exhilarating chapter.

Get ready to explore the secrets behind a metabolism that refuses to slow down, unlock the door to hormonal harmony, and fortify your bones with nutrition that whispers strength. We're not just here for a diet; we're here for a lifestyle revolution, one that celebrates the beauty and wisdom that come with age.

Within these pages, you'll find customizable plans, tantalizing recipes, and stories of resilience from real women who have embraced the Atkins approach and emerged victorious. It's time to shatter the stereotypes, redefine aging, and embrace the boundless potential that lies ahead.

So, if you're ready to step into a world where health meets vibrancy, where each day is a canvas waiting for your brushstroke, and where the Atkins Diet becomes your trusted ally in this thrilling journey – then buckle up. Your vibrant adventure begins now.

.

CHAPTER ONE
UNLEASHING YOUR METABOLIC MAGIC

Understanding Age-Related Metabolism Challenges

In the enchanting journey of life, one of the key companions that undergoes significant changes is our metabolism. As women gracefully step into their sixties, they often find themselves facing the mysterious slowdown of this vital bodily function. Understanding age-related metabolism challenges becomes imperative for those seeking to maintain a healthy weight and overall well-being.

Metabolism, the intricate process by which the body converts what you eat and drink into energy, tends to decelerate with age. This natural phenomenon can be attributed to various factors, including a decrease in muscle mass, hormonal fluctuations, and lifestyle changes. As we age, the body tends to lose muscle, which plays a pivotal role in supporting a higher metabolism. Hormonal changes, particularly during menopause, can further contribute to weight gain and a sluggish metabolism.

The Atkins Diet, designed to be a powerful ally in the battle against age-related metabolism challenges, addresses these issues head-on. By adopting a low-carb, high-protein approach, the diet aims to boost metabolism and facilitate effective weight management. Proteins, known as the building blocks of the body, become even more crucial in this stage of life. They aid in the preservation and building of lean muscle mass, countering the natural decline that often accompanies aging.

Moreover, the Atkins Diet recognizes the significance of healthy fats in the metabolic equation. Contrary to the outdated belief that all fats are detrimental, the diet emphasizes incorporating good fats that contribute to sustained energy and metabolic vitality. By understanding the nuanced needs of a mature metabolism, women over 60 can harness the power of the Atkins principles to reignite their metabolic magic.

Tailoring Atkins Principles to Boost Your Metabolism

Now that we've unveiled the metabolic challenges associated with aging, let's dive into the art of tailoring

Atkins principles to boost your metabolism effectively. The Atkins Diet, renowned for its success in weight management, becomes an even more potent tool when customized to meet the specific needs of women over 60.

At the core of the Atkins approach lies the reduction of carbohydrates, particularly those of the refined and processed variety. This strategic reduction serves multiple purposes, including stabilizing blood sugar levels and prompting the body to burn stored fat for energy. For women facing age-related metabolism challenges, this low-carb strategy is a game-changer.

Proteins take center stage in the Atkins Diet, and rightly so. Tailoring the intake of proteins to match the unique requirements of women over 60 contributes significantly to metabolic enhancement. Proteins not only support muscle preservation but also induce a thermic effect, meaning they require more energy to digest, thereby boosting the overall metabolic rate.

Simultaneously, the inclusion of healthy fats plays a pivotal role in the customization process. Avocados, nuts, and olive oil are not just indulgences; they are essential components that contribute to sustained energy levels and metabolic efficiency. The Atkins Diet encourages women to embrace these fats, understanding that they are not only delicious but also integral to the metabolic magic we seek to unleash.

Tailoring also extends beyond macronutrients to embrace micronutrients. Adequate intake of vitamins and minerals, especially those associated with metabolism like B-vitamins and iron, becomes a crucial part of the tailored Atkins plan. By aligning nutritional intake with the specific needs of women over 60, the diet becomes a personalized roadmap to metabolic rejuvenation.

The Atkins principles, when thoughtfully customized, act as a catalyst for metabolic transformation. It's not a one-size-fits-all approach; it's a bespoke journey that empowers women to take charge of their metabolism and, consequently, their overall health.

Overcoming Weight Loss Plateaus with Proven Strategies

Weight loss plateaus can be disheartening, especially when you're putting in the effort and not seeing the desired results. However, for women over 60 navigating the Atkins Diet, overcoming these plateaus is not just a possibility; it's a proven reality. Let's explore the strategies that serve as the secret weapons against stagnation in your weight loss journey.

Firstly, understanding the concept of a weight loss plateau is essential. It often occurs when the body adapts to the changes in diet and exercise, slowing down the rate of weight loss. This adaptive response can be particularly prevalent in those who have already shed a significant amount of weight. However, rest assured, overcoming this hurdle is not only possible but an integral part of the Atkins journey.

The Atkins Diet employs the concept of carb cycling as a potent strategy to break through plateaus. By strategically reintroducing slightly higher levels of carbohydrates at specific intervals, the body is kept from adapting to a consistent low-carb intake. This cycling approach not only prevents plateaus but also provides a welcome psychological break from the rigidity of a continuous low-carb diet.

Another proven strategy involves reevaluating your macronutrient intake. As your body changes, so do its nutritional needs. Periodically reassessing your protein, fat, and carbohydrate intake ensures that your diet aligns with your current metabolic requirements. The Atkins Diet, with its emphasis on flexibility and customization, allows women over 60 to tweak their macronutrient ratios to suit their evolving needs, preventing plateaus before they even appear.

Physical activity also plays a crucial role in overcoming weight loss plateaus. Introducing varied and challenging exercises, especially those that promote muscle development, can kickstart your metabolism and reignite the fat-burning process. The Atkins Diet encourages a holistic approach to well-being, recognizing that both nutrition and exercise are integral components of the weight loss journey.

The power of patience and persistence cannot be overstated. Weight loss plateaus are a natural part of the process, and breaking through them requires time and commitment. Celebrate the progress you've made, reassess your goals, and stay dedicated to the Atkins principles. Remember, it's not just about losing weight; it's about transforming your metabolism and embracing a healthier, more vibrant life.

Nutrient-Rich Foods

Hormonal Harmony: Navigating Menopause with Atkins

Hormones and Weight: A Delicate Balancing Act

As women gracefully enter the stage of menopause, they often find themselves embarking on a journey where hormonal fluctuations become a central theme. This chapter delves into the delicate balancing act between hormones and weight, shedding light on the profound impact that menopause can have on the body's composition and the role Atkins plays in harmonizing this intricate dance.

Menopause, a natural biological process, marks the end of a woman's reproductive years. It is characterized by a decline in estrogen and progesterone levels, leading to a variety of physical and emotional changes. One of the significant challenges many women face during this transition is weight gain, especially around the abdominal area. The delicate balance of hormones during menopause can contribute to increased fat storage and a slower metabolism.

Understanding the hormonal nuances during menopause is crucial for women seeking to manage their weight effectively. Estrogen, which plays a role in regulating metabolism, tends to decrease during menopause, potentially leading to weight gain. The decline in progesterone can also influence water retention and bloating, further complicating the weight management equation.

This delicate balancing act of hormones requires a tailored approach, and this is where the Atkins Diet steps in as a valuable ally. The low-carb, high-protein foundation of the Atkins principles becomes particularly relevant in the context of menopausal weight management. Proteins, known for their muscle-preserving properties, become essential in counteracting the natural loss of muscle mass that often accompanies hormonal changes.

Furthermore, the controlled carbohydrate intake advocated by the Atkins Diet helps stabilize blood sugar levels, preventing the spikes and crashes that can exacerbate hormonal imbalances. The diet's emphasis on healthy fats contributes to satiety and sustained energy, providing a stabilizing effect on mood and cravings.

By acknowledging the delicate balancing act between hormones and weight, women over 60 can embrace the Atkins approach to navigate this challenging terrain. The synergy between hormonal harmony and nutritional choices becomes a powerful tool in not only managing weight but also fostering overall well-being during the menopausal transition.

Atkins-Friendly Foods for Hormonal Stability

Navigating menopause is like traversing uncharted waters, and the foods we choose to consume can either be a source of turbulence or a steady sail through the hormonal storm. In this section, we explore the Atkins-friendly foods that contribute to hormonal stability, offering a delicious and practical roadmap for women over 60 seeking harmony during this transformative phase.

Proteins take center stage in the Atkins Diet, and their role in promoting hormonal stability cannot be overstated. During menopause, the preservation and building of muscle become essential for weight management and metabolic health. Incorporating lean proteins such as poultry, fish, tofu, and legumes provides the necessary amino acids to support muscle function and combat the natural decline in muscle mass associated with hormonal changes.

Healthy fats become the unsung heroes in the quest for hormonal stability. Avocados, nuts, seeds, and olive oil are not just culinary delights; they are rich sources of monounsaturated and polyunsaturated fats that play a crucial role in hormone production. These fats serve as precursors to hormones and contribute to the body's ability to synthesize and regulate hormones effectively.

Omega-3 fatty acids, found in fatty fish like salmon and trout, walnuts, and flaxseeds, are particularly beneficial during menopause. They have anti-inflammatory properties, which can help alleviate some of the common symptoms associated with hormonal fluctuations, such as joint pain and mood swings.

Low-carb vegetables become the nutritional powerhouses that provide a plethora of vitamins, minerals, and fiber without causing significant spikes in blood sugar. Broccoli, spinach, kale, and cauliflower are not only nutrient-dense but also contribute to a feeling of fullness, aiding in weight management and hormonal balance.

In addition to specific food choices, the timing and composition of meals play a vital role in hormonal stability. The Atkins Diet encourages a balanced distribution of macronutrients across meals, helping to regulate blood sugar levels throughout the day. This approach prevents the erratic spikes and crashes that can exacerbate hormonal imbalances and disrupt the delicate dance of hormones during menopause.

By incorporating these Atkins-friendly foods into their diet, women over 60 can proactively support hormonal stability. It's not just about what you eat; it's about choosing foods that become allies in the hormonal journey, paving the way for a smoother and more harmonious transition through menopause.

Tackling Menopausal Symptoms through Smart Nutrition

Menopause is a symphony of change, and the symptoms that accompany this phase can vary widely from woman to woman. Smart nutrition becomes a powerful tool in tackling these menopausal symptoms head-on, offering relief and support during a time of transformation. In this section, we explore how the Atkins Diet, with its focus on intelligent nutritional choices, becomes a beacon of hope for women navigating the seas of menopausal symptoms.

Hot flashes, mood swings, and sleep disturbances are common companions during menopause, and the foods we choose can either exacerbate or alleviate these symptoms. The Atkins Diet, with its emphasis on stable blood sugar levels, provides a foundation for managing mood swings and energy fluctuations. By avoiding refined carbohydrates and sugar, women over 60 can minimize the risk of blood sugar spikes and crashes, contributing to a more stable emotional state.

The inclusion of nutrient-dense foods in the Atkins approach becomes instrumental in addressing specific menopausal symptoms. Foods rich in calcium and vitamin D, such as dairy products, leafy greens, and fatty fish, contribute to bone health and can alleviate the risk of osteoporosis – a concern that often intensifies during menopause due to hormonal changes.

The relationship between nutrition and sleep is intricate, and during menopause, sleep disturbances can become more prevalent. The Atkins Diet recognizes the importance of magnesium in promoting relaxation and quality sleep. Magnesium-rich foods, including nuts, seeds, and dark leafy greens, become valuable additions to the diet, potentially easing sleep-related challenges.

The anti-inflammatory properties of certain foods, a hallmark of the Atkins Diet, can also play a role in managing joint pain and discomfort that may arise during menopause. Fatty fish, nuts, and olive oil, with their omega-3 fatty acids and other anti-inflammatory compounds, contribute to a more comfortable and active lifestyle.

Furthermore, hydration becomes a key component of smart nutrition during menopause. Adequate water intake can help alleviate symptoms like bloating and hot flashes, promoting overall well-being. The Atkins Diet, with its emphasis on whole, water-rich foods and mindful hydration, aligns with the holistic approach needed to tackle the multifaceted challenges of menopause.

Tackling menopausal symptoms through smart nutrition is not just about finding temporary relief; it's about cultivating a lifestyle that supports and enhances overall well-being. The Atkins Diet, with its science-backed principles and emphasis on intelligent food choices, becomes a compass guiding woman over 60 towards a smoother and more empowered journey through menopause.

CHAPTER THREE
BONES OF STEEL: STRENGTHENING YOUR FOUNDATION

The Role of Nutrition in Bone Health After 60

As we gracefully age, our bones undergo changes that require meticulous attention and care, especially for women over 60. This chapter delves into the critical role of nutrition in maintaining bone health, providing insights and strategies to ensure your foundation remains robust and resilient.

Bone health is a lifelong pursuit, and as we enter the golden years, it becomes increasingly vital to fortify our skeletal structure against the natural effects of aging. Bones are dynamic tissues that constantly undergo remodeling, with old bone being replaced by new bone. This process, known as bone turnover, tends to favor the creation of new bone during youth but gradually shifts towards a more balanced turnover in later years. For women, the onset of menopause adds another layer of complexity, as the decline in estrogen levels accelerates bone loss.

The foundation for strong and healthy bones is laid through proper nutrition, an aspect that becomes even more crucial after the age of 60. Calcium, the building block of bones, takes center stage in this nutritional symphony. While dairy products like milk and cheese are well-known sources of calcium, the Atkins Diet broadens the horizon by introducing alternative sources such as leafy greens, nuts, and fortified foods. This diversity ensures that even those with dietary restrictions or preferences can attain their recommended daily intake of calcium.

Vitamin D, the sunshine vitamin, plays a tandem role with calcium in bone health. It facilitates the absorption of calcium from the digestive system into the bloodstream and ensures its delivery to the bones. Women over 60 often face challenges in synthesizing vitamin D from sunlight due to factors like reduced sun exposure and decreased skin thickness. The Atkins Diet recognizes this and advocates for vitamin D-rich foods like fatty fish, eggs, and fortified products, providing a comprehensive approach to bone health.

Protein, another essential component of bone structure, is emphasized in the Atkins Diet for its role in preserving and building lean muscle mass. As bones and muscles share a dynamic relationship, maintaining muscle strength contributes to overall skeletal health. Protein-rich foods such as lean meats, poultry, and plant-based sources become not only sources of amino acids but also allies in the battle against age-related bone loss.

Phosphorus, often overshadowed by calcium, is equally crucial for bone health. These mineral forms a significant part of the bone structure, contributing to its strength and rigidity. The Atkins Diet, with its focus on a variety of protein sources, naturally incorporates phosphorus into the nutritional mix, offering a holistic approach to supporting bone density.

Magnesium, yet another unsung hero, plays a vital role in bone health by aiding in the activation of vitamin D and contributing to bone mineralization. Nuts, seeds, and leafy greens, staples of the Atkins Diet, are rich sources of magnesium, ensuring that your bones receive this often-overlooked nutrient.

The Atkins approach also addresses the delicate balance between acidic and alkaline foods. While the body requires a slightly alkaline environment for optimal bone health, a diet high in acidic foods can lead to calcium leaching from the bones. By promoting a balance between acidic and alkaline foods, the Atkins Diet contributes to the overall pH balance in the body, safeguarding against bone density loss.

In essence, the role of nutrition in bone health after 60 is a multifaceted endeavor. It involves not only ensuring an adequate intake of specific nutrients but also adopting a dietary approach that aligns with the dynamic needs of aging bones. The Atkins Diet, with its emphasis on a balanced and varied nutritional intake, emerges as a valuable ally in the quest for bones of steel.

Atkins Superfoods for Stronger Bones

Building on the foundational understanding of nutrition's pivotal role in bone health, let's explore the symphony of nutrients that Atkins superfoods bring to the stage, enhancing the strength and resilience of your bones. These superfoods go beyond meeting basic nutritional requirements, offering a symphony of essential elements that contribute to a robust skeletal foundation.

1. **Salmon: A Vitamin D Powerhouse**

    - Fatty fish, particularly salmon, takes the spotlight as a vitamin D powerhouse. Beyond its contribution to bone health, vitamin D is also recognized for its immune-boosting properties and potential mood-enhancing effects. Including salmon in your diet, as advocated by the Atkins approach, provides a delicious and nutritious solution to fortify your bones.

2. **Leafy Greens: Calcium-Rich Elegance**

    - Dark leafy greens, such as kale, spinach, and collard greens, are elegant contributors to bone health. Rich in calcium, these superfoods offer a nutrient-dense alternative for those who may be lactose intolerant or prefer plant-based options. The Atkins Diet encourages the inclusion of these leafy greens, ensuring that your bones receive the calcium they need to stay strong and resilient.

3. **Almonds: A Crunchy Source of Bone Support**

    - Almonds, with their delightful crunch and nutritional prowess, emerge as a superfood that supports bone health. Packed with calcium and magnesium, almonds provide a dynamic duo of nutrients essential for bone mineralization and overall skeletal strength. As a snack or a versatile ingredient in recipes, almonds add both flavor and nutritional value to your bone-friendly diet.

4. Greek Yogurt: Protein and Probiotics for Bone Resilience

- Greek yogurt, a protein-rich and probiotic-packed delight, earns its place as a superfood for bone resilience. High in calcium and phosphorus, Greek yogurt contributes to bone mineralization, while its probiotic content supports gut health. The Atkins Diet recognizes the importance of this dairy gem, offering a tasty and nutritious option for those on the quest for stronger bones.

5. Broccoli: A Versatile Cruciferous Ally

- Broccoli, part of the cruciferous vegetable family, emerges as a versatile ally in the journey to stronger bones. Beyond its calcium content, broccoli contains compounds that may have anti-inflammatory and antioxidant properties, contributing to overall bone health. The Atkins Diet encourages the incorporation of broccoli into various dishes, ensuring that you savor both taste and bone-nourishing benefits.

6. Eggs: Versatile and Vitamin D-Rich

- Eggs, a kitchen staple celebrated for their versatility, also offer a rich source of vitamin D. Supporting bone health while providing an array of essential nutrients, eggs become a convenient and nutritious addition to the Atkins Diet. Whether enjoyed scrambled, poached, or as part of a recipe, eggs contribute to the symphony of nutrients essential for stronger bones.

7. **Chia Seeds: Omega-3 Boost for Bone Density**

- Chia seeds, tiny powerhouses of nutrition, earn their place as an omega-3 boost for bone density. Rich in phosphorus, magnesium, and omega-3 fatty acids, these little seeds offer a nutritional punch that supports bone health. The Atkins Diet welcomes chia seeds into the dietary repertoire, allowing you to sprinkle bone-loving goodness into your meals.

These Atkins superfoods form a symphony of nutrients that not only meet the basic requirements for bone health but elevate the nutritional composition of your diet. By incorporating these superfoods into your meals, you not only fortify your bones but also indulge in a culinary experience that celebrates taste and well-being.

Crafting A Diet that Shields your Bones from Osteoporosis

Osteoporosis, a condition characterized by weakened and fragile bones, looms as a potential concern for many women as they age. Crafting a diet that shields your bones from osteoporosis becomes a proactive and empowering approach to prevent this condition. In this section, we explore the strategies advocated by the Atkins Diet to fortify your bones against the threat of osteoporosis.

1. **Strategic Calcium Intake**

   - The cornerstone of any diet aiming to shield bones from osteoporosis is strategic calcium intake. The Atkins Diet recognizes the significance of calcium in bone health and encourages the consumption of a variety of calcium-rich foods. This includes dairy products, leafy greens, fortified foods, and alternatives for those with specific dietary preferences. By strategically incorporating these sources, you create a robust foundation for bone resilience.

2. **Vitamin D Synergy**

   - Vitamin D, a synergistic partner to calcium, plays a pivotal role in preventing osteoporosis. The Atkins Diet, with its emphasis on vitamin D-rich foods like fatty fish, eggs, and fortified products, ensures that your bones receive the support they need. Additionally, sensible exposure to sunlight, a natural source of vitamin D, becomes part of the holistic approach advocated by Atkins for bone health.

3. Protein for Bone Preservation

- Protein, often associated with muscle health, also plays a crucial role in bone preservation. The Atkins Diet recognizes the intricate connection between bones and muscles, encouraging a protein-centric approach to support both. By preserving and building lean muscle mass through adequate protein intake, you contribute to the overall resilience of your skeletal structure.

4. Magnesium: The Silent Guardian

- Magnesium, often referred to as the silent guardian of bone health, deserves special attention in the prevention of osteoporosis. Nuts, seeds, and leafy greens, staples of the Atkins Diet, provide rich sources of magnesium. This mineral not only aids in bone mineralization but also supports overall muscle function, contributing to the dual benefit of bone and muscle health.

5. Balancing Alkalinity

- Crafting a diet that shields your bones from osteoporosis involves paying attention to the balance between acidic and alkaline foods. The Atkins Diet, with its emphasis on a balanced nutritional approach, naturally contributes to maintaining the body's overall pH balance. By avoiding excessive consumption of acidic foods, you prevent calcium leaching from the bones, supporting long-term bone health.

6. **Weight-Bearing Exercise: A Companion to Diet**

   - While diet forms a critical component in preventing osteoporosis, weight-bearing exercise stands as a companion in this endeavor. The Atkins Diet recognizes the importance of a holistic approach to bone health, encouraging physical activity that includes weight-bearing exercises. This combination of a bone-friendly diet and regular exercise becomes a powerful strategy to shield your bones from the impact of osteoporosis.

7. **Avoiding Excessive Alcohol and Caffeine**

   - Excessive alcohol and caffeine intake can contribute to bone loss and increase the risk of osteoporosis. The Atkins Diet, with its emphasis on mindful nutrition, advocates for moderation in the consumption of these beverages. By being conscious of your alcohol and caffeine intake, you contribute to the overall protection of your bones against potential risk factors.

Crafting a diet that shields your bones from osteoporosis involves a thoughtful and comprehensive approach. The Atkins Diet, with its focus on strategic nutrient intake, balanced alkalinity, and holistic well-being, emerges as a valuable ally in this journey. By adopting these strategies into your lifestyle, you not only fortify your bones against osteoporosis but also embrace a proactive and empowering stance toward your long-term bone health.

CHAPTER FOUR
POWERING UP: BUILDING AND PRESERVING MUSCLE MASS

Protein-Packed Perfection: Your Muscle's Best Friend

Muscles are the engine that propels us through life, and as we age, preserving and building muscle mass becomes a paramount concern. This section explores the role of protein, the muscle's best friend, in powering up your physique, and how the Atkins Diet provides a protein-packed perfection formula for muscular vitality.

Protein, often hailed as the building block of life, is especially crucial in the context of muscle health. As we age, the natural process of muscle protein synthesis diminishes, making the preservation and augmentation of muscle mass an essential aspect of healthy aging. The Atkins Diet, with its emphasis on a high-protein approach, stands as an ideal companion in the quest for protein-packed perfection and robust muscles.

The primary components of muscle, amino acids, are derived from protein. Adequate protein intake provides the body with these essential building blocks, supporting the repair and regeneration of muscle tissue. For women over 60, who may face challenges related to age-related muscle loss, protein becomes a vital ally in maintaining strength and functionality.

The Atkins Diet recommends a protein-centric approach, advocating for a variety of protein sources to ensure a comprehensive amino acid profile. Lean meats, poultry, fish, eggs, and plant-based proteins like tofu and legumes become staples, offering diverse options to meet individual preferences and dietary needs. By incorporating these protein-packed foods into your meals, you not only support muscle health but also enjoy a varied and satisfying diet.

Moreover, the Atkins approach goes beyond quantity to emphasize the quality of protein. Choosing lean, high-quality protein sources ensures that you not only meet your protein requirements but also avoid unnecessary saturated fats and additives. This quality-focused perspective aligns with the overall goal of promoting health and well-being through a balanced and nutritious diet.

In essence, protein is the key to muscle-packing perfection, and the Atkins Diet provides a blueprint for achieving this perfection. By making protein a central focus of your dietary intake, you empower your muscles to stay strong, resilient, and ready to take on the challenges of life.

Resistance Training and The Atkins Diet: A Dynamic Duo

While protein lays the foundation for muscle health, the synergy between resistance training and the Atkins Diet creates a dynamic duo that elevates your journey to building and preserving muscle mass. In this section, we delve into the profound impact of resistance training and how it harmonizes with the principles of the Atkins Diet for a muscular vitality boost.

Resistance training, commonly known as strength or weight training, involves working against a force to build muscle strength, endurance, and size. This form of exercise becomes increasingly significant as we age, as it directly addresses the age-related decline in muscle mass and function. The Atkins Diet recognizes the importance of resistance training and encourages its integration into a holistic approach to muscular vitality.

One of the key benefits of resistance training is its ability to stimulate muscle protein synthesis, the process by which the body builds new muscle proteins. This stimulation becomes particularly crucial for women over 60, who may experience a natural decline in muscle protein synthesis. By engaging in resistance training, you not only counteract this decline but also promote the growth and preservation of lean muscle mass.

The synergy between resistance training and the high-protein approach of the Atkins Diet becomes a potent formula for muscle-building success. Protein provides the necessary amino acids for muscle repair and growth, while resistance training creates the stimulus for the body to utilize these amino acids effectively. Together, they form a dynamic duo that accelerates the pace of muscle development and fortifies your physique.

Moreover, resistance training contributes to improvements in overall strength, balance, and functionality – essential elements for maintaining an active and independent lifestyle. The Atkins Diet, aligning with the holistic philosophy of well-being, recognizes the multidimensional benefits of resistance training beyond muscle building. By incorporating this dynamic duo into your routine, you not only sculpt a more muscular physique but also enhance your overall physical capabilities.

The Atkins approach also addresses the nutritional needs associated with resistance training. Adequate protein intake, coupled with the controlled intake of carbohydrates, ensures that your body has the necessary fuel for both muscle-building and recovery. This balanced nutritional approach aligns with the principles of the Atkins Diet, creating a seamless integration between diet and exercise for optimal results.

In conclusion, resistance training and the Atkins Diet form a dynamic duo that transcends the conventional boundaries of muscle-building strategies. By harmonizing the principles of high-quality protein intake with the stimulating effects of resistance training, you unlock a powerful synergy that not only transforms your physique but also enhances your overall strength and vitality.

Staying Strong and Active - Your Guide To Muscular Vitality

Staying strong and active well into the golden years is a universal aspiration, and achieving muscular vitality becomes a key component of this journey. In this section, we explore the holistic guide provided by the Atkins Diet for maintaining muscular strength, functionality, and an active lifestyle.

1. **Balanced Nutrition for Muscle Preservation**

   - The foundation of muscular vitality lies in balanced nutrition, and the Atkins Diet serves as a comprehensive guide for achieving this balance. Protein, the cornerstone of muscle health, takes center stage, ensuring that your muscles receive the essential amino acids for repair and growth. The diet's emphasis on high-quality protein sources, coupled with a controlled intake of carbohydrates, creates an optimal nutritional environment for muscle preservation.

2. **Resistance Training: A Lifelong Companion**

   - As we age, the importance of resistance training becomes increasingly evident. The Atkins Diet, aligning with the holistic philosophy of well-being, encourages resistance training as a lifelong companion for maintaining muscular vitality. Engaging in regular strength or weight training exercises not only builds and preserves muscle mass but also enhances bone density, joint health, and overall functional capacity.

3. **Hydration and Electrolyte Balance**

- Muscular vitality is not only about strength but also about ensuring that your muscles function optimally. Adequate hydration and electrolyte balance, integral components of the Atkins approach, play a vital role in muscle function. Staying hydrated supports nutrient transport to muscle cells, while electrolytes like potassium and sodium contribute to muscle contraction and relaxation. This holistic approach to muscle health ensures that your muscles remain vital and responsive.

4. **Adequate Rest and Recovery**

- In the pursuit of muscular vitality, recognizing the importance of rest and recovery is paramount. The Atkins Diet, emphasizing a balanced and sustainable lifestyle, acknowledges the significance of giving your muscles the time they need to repair and grow. Quality sleep, stress management, and allowing adequate recovery between resistance training sessions become integral components of the guide to muscular vitality.

5. **Mind-Body Connection**

- The Atkins approach transcends the physical aspects of muscle health and acknowledges the mind-body connection. Mental well-being, stress reduction, and mindfulness contribute to a holistic guide for maintaining muscular vitality. By incorporating practices like meditation, yoga, or other forms of relaxation into your routine, you enhance the overall well-being of both your body and mind, creating a harmonious environment for muscular health.

6. **Lifelong Learning and Adaptation**

- Muscular vitality is not a static goal but a dynamic journey that requires lifelong learning and adaptation. The Atkins Diet, with its emphasis on flexibility and customization, aligns with this philosophy. As your body evolves, so do its nutritional and exercise needs. The guide to muscular vitality provided by the Atkins approach encourages continuous learning, adaptation, and a proactive stance toward optimizing your muscle health.

In essence, staying strong and active is not a destination but a continuous exploration, and the Atkins Diet serves as a valuable guide for this journey. By embracing a balanced nutritional approach, incorporating resistance training, prioritizing hydration and recovery, nurturing the mind-body connection, and fostering a mindset of lifelong learning, you empower yourself to enjoy the benefits of muscular vitality well into the tapestry of your life.

Carbs and Blood Sugar: Navigating the Connection

Understanding the intricate dance between carbohydrates and blood sugar is pivotal for effective diabetes defense. This section explores the connection between carbs and blood sugar, shedding light on the role Atkins plays in navigating this delicate balance and providing a robust defense against diabetes.

The Carbohydrate Conundrum: Impact on Blood Sugar

Carbohydrates, often referred to as the body's primary source of energy, play a central role in the regulation of blood sugar levels. When consumed, carbohydrates are broken down into glucose (sugar), which enters the bloodstream. The rise in blood glucose triggers the pancreas to release insulin, a hormone that facilitates the uptake of glucose by cells for energy or storage.

For individuals with diabetes, this process can become disrupted. In type 2 diabetes, the body's cells may become resistant to the action of insulin, leading to elevated blood sugar levels. In type 1 diabetes, the pancreas produces little to no insulin, causing a similar imbalance. Navigating the connection between carbs and blood sugar becomes a crucial aspect of diabetes management and prevention.

Atkins and the Low-Carb Advantage

The Atkins Diet, renowned for its low-carbohydrate approach, becomes a powerful ally in the quest for blood sugar control. By restricting the intake of high-carb foods, Atkins helps regulate blood sugar levels, minimizing the spikes and crashes that can pose challenges for individuals with diabetes.

The diet's emphasis on low-carb, high-fat, and moderate-protein intake aims to achieve a state of ketosis. In ketosis, the body shifts its primary fuel source from glucose to ketones, which are derived from fats. This metabolic state can have profound effects on blood sugar regulation. By reducing reliance on glucose, Atkins minimizes the impact of carbohydrates on blood sugar, offering a strategic defense against diabetes.

The Glycemic Impact: Different Carbs, Different Effects

Not all carbohydrates are created equal, and their glycemic impact varies based on factors such as type and fiber content. Atkins recognizes the nuances of the glycemic index, a scale that measures how quickly a carbohydrate-containing food raises blood sugar levels. By favoring low-glycemic foods, Atkins provides a roadmap for navigating the connection between carbs and blood sugar.

Low-glycemic foods, such as non-starchy vegetables, nuts, and seeds, have a slower impact on blood sugar, promoting more stable levels. In contrast, high-glycemic foods, like refined sugars and grains, can lead to rapid spikes in blood sugar. The Atkins approach guides individuals towards carb choices that align with the principles of blood sugar control, offering a nuanced strategy for diabetes defense.

Balancing Macros for Blood Sugar Stability

Beyond carb reduction, the Atkins Diet emphasizes a balanced distribution of macronutrients – carbohydrates, proteins, and fats – to promote blood sugar stability. Protein, with its minimal impact on blood sugar, becomes a crucial component in maintaining satiety and preventing excessive carb intake. Healthy fats contribute to a feeling of fullness, further supporting blood sugar control by reducing the likelihood of overeating.

By orchestrating this balance, Atkins creates a nutritional symphony that harmonizes with the body's natural mechanisms for blood sugar regulation. The controlled intake of carbohydrates, coupled with an optimal distribution of macronutrients, establishes a foundation for stable blood sugar levels, forming a robust defense against the progression and complications of diabetes.

Personalizing Carb Intake: Individualized Diabetes Defense

Recognizing that individuals vary in their response to carbohydrates, the Atkins Diet embraces a personalized approach to diabetes defense. The concept of 'Net Carbs,' which subtracts fiber content from total carbs, allows for a more tailored approach to carb intake. This personalized strategy accommodates individual preferences, dietary needs, and the nuances of blood sugar management.

Furthermore, Atkins acknowledges the role of individual tolerance for carbohydrates. Some individuals may thrive with a slightly higher carb intake, while others may benefit from stricter carb control. This flexibility empowers individuals with diabetes to fine-tune their dietary approach, fostering a sense of control and ownership in their diabetes defense.

Long-Term Benefits: Beyond Blood Sugar Control

The advantages of navigating the connection between carbs and blood sugar extend beyond immediate glucose management. The Atkins Diet, as part of a comprehensive diabetes defense strategy, offers long-term benefits that contribute to overall health and well-being.

Weight management, often intertwined with diabetes management, is a key focus of the Atkins approach. By promoting satiety, stabilizing blood sugar, and encouraging the utilization of stored fat for energy, Atkins becomes a sustainable solution for weight control – a factor that significantly impacts diabetes progression and complications.

Inflammation, a common concern in individuals with diabetes, is also addressed by the anti-inflammatory effects of the Atkins Diet. By emphasizing whole, nutrient-dense foods and minimizing the intake of processed and inflammatory foods, Atkins supports an environment that mitigates inflammation, contributing to enhanced overall health.

Therefore, navigating the connection between carbs and blood sugar is at the heart of effective diabetes defense. The Atkins Diet, with its low-carbohydrate, balanced macronutrient approach, offers a strategic and personalized defense against the challenges posed by diabetes. By understanding the impact of carbs on blood sugar, embracing a glycemic-conscious mindset, and incorporating long-term health benefits, Atkins becomes a holistic and empowering ally in the journey towards blood sugar control and optimal well-being.

Crafting Low-Carb Meals for Stable Blood Sugar

Crafting low-carb meals forms the cornerstone of the Atkins approach to diabetes defense. The fundamental principle is to limit the intake of carbohydrates, especially those with a high glycemic impact, to regulate blood sugar levels effectively. By understanding the low-carb approach, individuals with diabetes can navigate their culinary choices with precision, creating meals that not only delight the taste buds but also contribute to stable blood sugar.

Atkins categorizes carbohydrates into three main groups: Net Carbs, Foundation Vegetables, and High-Carb Vegetables. Net Carbs are calculated by subtracting fiber content from total carbs, offering a more accurate representation of a food's impact on blood sugar. Foundation Vegetables, low in Net Carbs, form the basis of the diet, providing essential nutrients without causing significant spikes in blood sugar. High-Carb Vegetables, with a higher Net Carb content, are introduced gradually and in controlled portions.

Building the Foundation: Incorporating Foundation Vegetables

Foundation Vegetables, rich in fiber and low in Net Carbs, play a pivotal role in crafting low-carb meals that support stable blood sugar levels. These vegetables include leafy greens like spinach and kale, cruciferous vegetables like broccoli and cauliflower, and other nutrient-dense options such as zucchini and bell peppers.

One of the advantages of incorporating Foundation Vegetables is their versatility. From salads to stir-fries, these vegetables can be featured in a variety of dishes, adding color, flavor, and nutritional value. The fiber content in these vegetables contributes to satiety, helping individuals feel full and satisfied without experiencing rapid spikes in blood sugar.

Crafting a low-carb meal with Foundation Vegetables often involves exploring creative cooking methods. Roasting, sautéing, and grilling can enhance the natural flavors of these vegetables, making them a delicious and satisfying component of any dish. By building the foundation of a meal with nutrient-dense and low-carb vegetables, individuals with diabetes lay the groundwork for stable blood sugar control.

Protein Power: The Heart of Low-Carb Meals

Protein takes center stage in crafting low-carb meals for stable blood sugar. Whether from animal or plant sources, protein is a macronutrient that has minimal impact on blood sugar levels. Including adequate protein in meals not only supports blood sugar stability but also contributes to muscle preservation, satiety, and overall well-being.

Lean meats, poultry, fish, eggs, tofu, and legumes are excellent sources of protein that can be featured in low-carb meals. Grilled chicken, salmon fillets, scrambled eggs with vegetables, or a hearty lentil soup are examples of protein-rich dishes that align with the principles of blood sugar control. The variety of protein options allows for diverse and enjoyable low-carb meal choices.

Balancing protein intake is essential, and the Atkins approach encourages individuals to choose a variety of protein sources while being mindful of portion sizes. By incorporating protein into each meal, individuals can create a satisfying and blood sugar-friendly culinary experience that supports their diabetes defense strategy.

Healthy Fats: Elevating Flavor and Satiety

Healthy fats play a crucial role in crafting low-carb meals that are not only nutritious but also flavorful and satisfying. While fats are dense in calories, they have a minimal impact on blood sugar levels. Including sources of healthy fats, such as avocados, olive oil, nuts, and seeds, adds richness and complexity to low-carb dishes.

One of the advantages of healthy fats is their ability to enhance the taste and texture of meals. A drizzle of olive oil on roasted vegetables, avocado slices in a salad, or a sprinkle of nuts on yogurt are examples of how healthy fats can elevate the culinary experience. By incorporating these fats into low-carb meals, individuals with diabetes create a sensorial journey that goes beyond the limitations of traditional dietary approaches.

Furthermore, healthy fats contribute to satiety, helping individuals feel full and satisfied after meals. This feeling of fullness can prevent overeating and snacking, contributing to overall blood sugar control. The Atkins Diet advocates for a balanced distribution of macronutrients, including healthy fats, to create meals that are not only blood sugar-friendly but also enjoyable and sustainable.

Smart Carb Choices: Introducing High-Carb Vegetables

While the low-carb approach forms the foundation of diabetes defense, Atkins recognizes that not all carbohydrates need to be strictly avoided. High-Carb Vegetables, introduced gradually and in controlled portions, expand the variety of flavors and textures in low-carb meals. These vegetables, such as sweet potatoes, carrots, and peas, offer nutritional benefits while still aligning with blood sugar control.

Incorporating High-Carb Vegetables requires a thoughtful and measured approach. Portion control is key, and individuals can experiment to find the right balance that works for their blood sugar management. Whether roasted as a side dish or blended into soups, these vegetables add a touch of sweetness and diversity to low-carb meals.

Balancing the inclusion of High-Carb Vegetables with the foundational principles of the Atkins Diet allows individuals with diabetes to customize their meals based on their preferences and nutritional needs. This nuanced approach creates a sustainable and flexible low-carb culinary experience that goes beyond restrictive diets, empowering individuals to enjoy a rich and varied diet while maintaining stable blood sugar levels.

Meal Planning for Success: Practical Tips and Recipes

Meal planning is a practical and empowering aspect of crafting low-carb meals for stable blood sugar. By approaching meals with intention and foresight, individuals can create a repertoire of recipes that align with their diabetes defense goals. The Atkins Diet provides practical tips and delicious recipes that cater to a low-carb lifestyle, making the process of meal planning both accessible and enjoyable.

Practical Tips for Crafting Low-Carb Meals:

1. **Variety is Key:** Incorporate a diverse range of vegetables, proteins, and healthy fats to create meals that are visually appealing and nutritionally balanced.

2. **Experiment with Herbs and Spices:** Enhance the flavor of low-carb dishes with a variety of herbs and spices. Experimenting with different seasonings adds

depth and excitement to meals without relying on excessive salt or sugar.

3. **Portion Control:** Be mindful of portion sizes, especially when including High-Carb Vegetables. Paying attention to portions helps manage overall carb intake and supports blood sugar control.

4. **Preparation is Half the Battle:** Plan and prepare meals in advance to avoid last-minute temptations or compromises. Having pre-prepared low-carb options readily available contributes to dietary success.

5. **Hydration Matters:** Stay hydrated throughout the day. Water not only supports overall health but also helps manage appetite and prevents overeating during meals.

6. **Enjoy the Process:** Embrace the journey of crafting low-carb meals as an opportunity for culinary exploration. Enjoying the process makes the commitment to blood sugar-friendly eating sustainable and rewarding.

Delicious Low-Carb Recipes for Inspiration:

1. **Grilled Lemon Herb Chicken with Roasted Asparagus:** Marinate chicken breasts in a mixture of lemon, herbs, and olive oil, then grill to perfection. Serve alongside roasted asparagus for a flavorful and low-carb meal.

2. **Zucchini Noodles with Pesto and Cherry Tomatoes:** Spiralize zucchini into noodles and toss with homemade pesto and cherry tomatoes. This refreshing dish is not only low in carbs but also bursting with fresh flavors.

3. **Mediterranean Salad with Feta and Olives:** Create a vibrant salad with mixed greens, cherry tomatoes, cucumber, feta cheese, and olives. Drizzle with olive oil and balsamic vinegar for a satisfying and blood sugar-friendly meal.

4. **Cauliflower Fried Rice with Shrimp:** Transform cauliflower rice into a delicious fried rice alternative by stir-frying with shrimp, vegetables, and a touch of soy sauce. This low-carb version of a classic dish is both satisfying and nutritious.

5. **Baked Salmon with Avocado Salsa:** Season salmon fillets with herbs and bake until flaky. Top with a refreshing salsa made from ripe avocados, cherry tomatoes, and cilantro for a nutrient-packed and low-carb meal.

Crafting low-carb meals for stable blood sugar is not just a dietary choice; it's a powerful strategy for diabetes defense. By understanding the principles of the low-carb approach, incorporating Foundation Vegetables, prioritizing protein and healthy fats, introducing High-Carb Vegetables in moderation, and embracing practical meal planning, individuals with diabetes can take control of their culinary choices.

The Atkins Diet serves as a guiding light in this journey, providing not only a framework for low-carb living but also a wealth of practical tips and delicious recipes. By adopting a flexible and enjoyable approach to low-carb eating, individuals with diabetes can experience the pleasure of varied and flavorful meals while safeguarding their blood sugar levels.

In essence, crafting low-carb meals for stable blood sugar is an act of empowerment. It's a declaration that individuals with diabetes can take charge of their dietary choices, savoring the richness of a diverse and satisfying culinary experience while nurturing their overall health and well-being. In this culinary exploration, the kitchen becomes a sanctuary where diabetes defense is not just a necessity but a celebration of the joy that comes with mindful and intentional eating.

The Atkins Approach to Diabetes Prevention and Management

Understanding the Diabetes Epidemic: A Call to Action

The global surge in diabetes prevalence calls for urgent attention and proactive measures. Diabetes, characterized by elevated blood sugar levels, poses significant health risks and complications if left unmanaged. The Atkins Diet, renowned for its low-carbohydrate approach, emerges as a strategic ally in the prevention and management of diabetes.

The diabetes epidemic is multifaceted, encompassing both type 1 and type 2 diabetes. While type 1 diabetes involves the immune system attacking and destroying insulin-producing cells, type 2 diabetes is largely associated with insulin resistance, where the body's cells become less responsive to insulin. The rise in type 2 diabetes, often linked to lifestyle factors including diet, highlights the need for targeted interventions that address the root causes of the condition.

Foundations of the Atkins Approach: Low-Carb Living for Blood Sugar Control

At the heart of the Atkins approach to diabetes prevention and management is the principle of low-carb living. The diet advocates for a reduction in carbohydrate intake, especially those with a high glycemic impact. By minimizing the consumption of foods that quickly raise blood sugar levels, individuals can better control their glucose levels, mitigating the risk of diabetes and supporting its management.

Carbohydrates, the primary source of glucose, are classified into three main categories within the Atkins framework: Net Carbs, Foundation Vegetables, and High-Carb Vegetables. Net Carbs represent the total carbs minus fiber content, providing a more accurate reflection of a food's impact on blood sugar. Foundation Vegetables, low in Net Carbs, form the basis of the diet, offering essential nutrients without causing significant blood sugar spikes. High-Carb Vegetables, introduced gradually and in controlled portions, expand the variety of flavors and textures in the diet.

The Atkins approach acknowledges that one size does not fit all, emphasizing a personalized and flexible strategy. Individuals can tailor their carbohydrate intake based on their unique needs, preferences, and health goals. This individualized approach fosters sustainability, empowering individuals to adopt a low-carb lifestyle that aligns with their diabetes prevention or management journey.

Blood Sugar Stability: The Key to Diabetes Defense

At the core of the Atkins approach to diabetes prevention and management is the concept of blood sugar stability. Unstable blood sugar levels, characterized by frequent spikes and crashes, contribute to insulin resistance and the progression of diabetes. By adopting a low-carb lifestyle, individuals aim to achieve and maintain stable blood sugar levels, providing a foundation for diabetes defense.

High-carbohydrate diets, especially those rich in refined sugars and grains, can lead to rapid spikes in blood sugar. These spikes trigger the release of insulin, contributing to insulin resistance over time. The Atkins approach, with its focus on low-carb living, minimizes the impact of carbohydrates on blood sugar, creating an environment conducive to stable glucose levels.

Stable blood sugar levels offer a range of health benefits beyond diabetes prevention and management. Individuals may experience increased energy levels, improved mental clarity, and reduced cravings for sugary foods. The Atkins approach promotes a sustained and balanced release of energy, preventing the energy highs and lows associated with fluctuations in blood sugar.

The Role of Ketosis in Diabetes Defense

Ketosis, a metabolic state where the body utilizes ketones derived from fats as a primary fuel source, plays a pivotal role in the Atkins approach to diabetes defense. By reducing reliance on glucose, the body can achieve and maintain ketosis, offering unique advantages for blood sugar control and overall health.

In ketosis, the body becomes efficient at burning stored fat for energy, contributing to weight management – a crucial factor in diabetes prevention and management. Excess body weight, especially abdominal fat, is linked to insulin resistance and an increased risk of type 2 diabetes. The Atkins approach addresses this connection by promoting fat utilization as a primary energy source, aiding in weight loss and maintenance.

Furthermore, ketones produced during ketosis serve as an alternative fuel for the brain, supporting cognitive function and mental clarity. This is particularly relevant for individuals with diabetes, as diabetes-related complications can include cognitive impairment. The Atkins approach, by harnessing the benefits of ketosis, provides a multifaceted defense against diabetes and its associated health risks.

Balanced Macronutrients for Comprehensive Diabetes Defense

While the low-carb aspect is central to the Atkins approach, it also emphasizes the importance of balanced macronutrients – proteins, fats, and carbohydrates – for comprehensive diabetes defense. Proteins and healthy fats play critical roles in blood sugar stability, satiety, and overall well-being.

Protein, with its minimal impact on blood sugar, is a key component in maintaining muscle mass and supporting metabolic health. The Atkins approach encourages the inclusion of a variety of protein sources, including lean meats, poultry, fish, eggs, tofu, and legumes. Adequate protein intake is essential for individuals with diabetes to prevent muscle loss, support satiety, and contribute to overall metabolic function.

Healthy fats, another crucial macronutrient, offer a range of benefits in the context of diabetes prevention and management. By incorporating sources such as avocados, olive oil, nuts, and seeds, individuals can enhance the flavor of meals, promote satiety, and contribute to stable blood sugar levels. The balanced distribution of macronutrients within the Atkins approach creates a sustainable and enjoyable dietary framework that aligns with diabetes defense goals.

Customization for Individual Needs: A Personalized Approach

Recognizing that individuals have unique needs and responses to dietary interventions; the Atkins approach embraces a personalized strategy for diabetes defense. The concept of 'Net Carbs,' which considers fiber content when calculating carbohydrate intake, allows for a more tailored approach to carb consumption. This customization accommodates individual preferences, dietary restrictions, and the nuances of blood sugar management.

Additionally, the Atkins approach acknowledges that individuals may have varying tolerances for carbohydrates. Some may thrive with a slightly higher carb intake, while others may benefit from stricter carb control. This flexibility empowers individuals to fine-tune their dietary approach based on their specific health goals, making diabetes defense a personalized and achievable endeavor.

Long-Term Benefits Beyond Diabetes Defense

Adopting the Atkins approach to diabetes prevention and management offers a spectrum of long-term benefits that extend beyond blood sugar control. Weight management, a critical factor in diabetes, is addressed through the promotion of fat utilization and the emphasis on satiating proteins and healthy fats. The Atkins approach becomes a sustainable solution for individuals seeking not only diabetes defense but also a pathway to overall well-being.

Inflammation, often elevated in individuals with diabetes, is also addressed by the anti-inflammatory effects of the Atkins Diet. The emphasis on whole, nutrient-dense foods and the reduction of processed and inflammatory foods contribute to an environment that mitigates inflammation, supporting cardiovascular health and longevity.

Moreover, the Atkins approach recognizes the interconnectedness of physical and mental well-being. Stable blood sugar levels, achieved through low-carb living, can positively impact mood, cognitive function, and overall mental health. By fostering a holistic approach to health, the Atkins Diet becomes a comprehensive strategy for individuals looking to safeguard their well-being in the long term.

Practical Tips for Integrating the Atkins Approach into Everyday Life

Implementing the Atkins approach into everyday life requires practical and actionable steps. Whether individuals are embarking on diabetes prevention or managing an existing condition, the following tips can guide them on their journey:

1. **Educate Yourself:** Gain a thorough understanding of the principles behind the Atkins approach and how it aligns with diabetes defense. Knowledge empowers individuals to make informed choices and navigate their dietary journey with confidence.

2. **Gradual Transition:** If transitioning to a low-carb lifestyle, consider making gradual changes to allow the body to adapt. Gradual adjustments can ease the process and prevent overwhelming changes.

3. **Embrace Variety:** Explore a diverse range of low-carb foods to keep meals interesting and enjoyable. Embracing variety ensures a well-rounded and nutritionally rich diet.

4. **Stay Hydrated:** Adequate hydration is essential for overall health and can support the body's natural processes, including blood sugar regulation. Aim to consume an appropriate amount of water throughout the day.

5. **Monitor Blood Sugar Levels:** Individuals with diabetes should regularly monitor their blood sugar levels to track the impact of dietary changes. This information can guide adjustments and ensure personalized diabetes defense.

6. **Incorporate Physical Activity:** Pairing the Atkins approach with regular physical activity enhances the benefits of diabetes defense. Exercise contributes to weight management, improves insulin sensitivity, and supports overall metabolic health.

7. **Consult with Healthcare Professionals:** Before making significant dietary changes, especially for individuals with diabetes or other health conditions, consulting with healthcare professionals is crucial. Healthcare providers can offer personalized guidance based on individual health needs.

Empowering Lives Through Diabetes Defense

The Atkins approach to diabetes prevention and management transcends conventional dietary strategies. It is a lifestyle framework that empowers individuals to take control of their health, defend against the challenges of diabetes, and embrace a pathway to long-term well-being.

By understanding the foundations of the Atkins approach, embracing blood sugar stability, harnessing the benefits of ketosis, balancing macronutrients, customizing for individual needs, and appreciating the long-term benefits, individuals can embark on a journey that extends beyond diabetes defense. The Atkins Diet becomes a companion in the holistic pursuit of health, offering practical tips and a flexible approach that accommodates the diverse needs and goals of individuals.

In essence, the Atkins approach to diabetes prevention and management is an invitation to a life of empowerment. It is a declaration that individuals have the agency to shape their health destiny, make choices that resonate with their unique selves, and enjoy the richness of a life lived in balance. Through diabetes defense, the Atkins approach becomes a beacon, guiding individuals towards a future where well-being is not just a goal but a lived reality.

CHAPTER SIX
BEYOND THE SCALE: HOLISTIC HEALTH FOR WOMEN OVER 60

Mental Clarity and Cognitive Boosts on the Atkins Diet

Unlocking the Mind-Body Connection

In the pursuit of holistic health for women over 60, mental clarity and cognitive function emerge as pivotal aspects that extend far beyond physical well-being. The mind-body connection is a profound and intricate relationship, and the Atkins Diet, renowned for its impact on weight management and metabolic health, also holds the potential to unleash cognitive benefits that contribute to mental clarity and overall brain function.

The Role of Nutrition in Cognitive Health

Understanding the interplay between nutrition and cognitive health is essential for women over 60 seeking to optimize mental clarity. The brain, a highly metabolically active organ, relies on a steady supply of nutrients for optimal function. Key components such as omega-3 fatty acids, antioxidants, vitamins, and minerals play crucial roles in supporting cognitive processes, memory, and overall brain health.

The Atkins Diet, with its emphasis on a balanced intake of macronutrients and nutrient-dense foods, aligns with the principles of brain-friendly nutrition. By prioritizing high-quality proteins, healthy fats, and a variety of vegetables, the diet lays the foundation for providing the brain with the essential nutrients it needs to thrive.

Blood Sugar Stability and Cognitive Performance

One of the fundamental tenets of the Atkins Diet is blood sugar stability. The impact of blood sugar levels on cognitive performance is well-documented, especially in the context of aging. Fluctuations in blood sugar can lead to energy crashes and contribute to cognitive fog, making stable blood sugar levels a key factor in maintaining mental clarity.

The low-carbohydrate approach of the Atkins Diet plays a significant role in blood sugar stability. By reducing the intake of high-glycemic carbohydrates that can cause rapid spikes and crashes in blood sugar, the diet supports a more consistent and sustained energy supply to the brain. This, in turn, contributes to enhanced cognitive function, improved focus, and sustained mental energy for women over 60.

Ketosis and Brain Fuel

The Atkins Diet's unique ability to induce ketosis becomes a notable player in the quest for mental clarity. Ketosis is a metabolic state where the body shifts from relying on glucose to utilizing ketones, which are produced from the breakdown of fats. The brain, despite its preference for glucose, can efficiently utilize ketones as an alternative fuel source.

Studies suggest that ketones may offer neuroprotective benefits and support cognitive function. The production of ketones during ketosis is associated with improved mitochondrial function, reduced oxidative stress, and enhanced production of brain-derived neurotrophic factor (BDNF), a protein crucial for cognitive processes and neuronal health.

While the brain can adapt to using ketones, the Atkins Diet's induction of ketosis may provide women over 60 with an additional avenue to support cognitive health. This metabolic flexibility, where the brain can seamlessly switch between glucose and ketones, showcases the intricate ways in which the Atkins Diet goes beyond weight management to impact overall well-being.

Antioxidants and Brain Defense

The inclusion of antioxidant-rich foods within the Atkins Diet adds another layer of support for cognitive health. Antioxidants, found in abundance in fruits, vegetables, and certain fats, play a crucial role in protecting the brain from oxidative stress and inflammation, both of which are implicated in age-related cognitive decline.

While the Atkins Diet limits the intake of high-carb fruits, it encourages the consumption of low-carb, antioxidant-rich vegetables such as leafy greens, bell peppers, and broccoli. Additionally, fats like olive oil and avocados, permitted on the diet, contribute to antioxidant defenses. These brain-protective antioxidants help neutralize free radicals and mitigate the cumulative damage that can impact cognitive function over time.

Omega-3 Fatty Acids and Brain Vitality

Omega-3 fatty acids, particularly EPA (eicosapentaenoic acid) and DHA (docosahexaenoic acid), are essential components for maintaining brain vitality. These fatty acids are integral to the structure of cell membranes in the brain and have been associated with improved cognitive function, memory, and mood.

While the Atkins Diet restricts the intake of certain high-carb fish, it allows for the consumption of fish rich in omega-3 fatty acids, such as salmon and mackerel. These fatty fish not only contribute to the overall macronutrient balance but also provide women over 60 with a source of these critical brain-boosting fatty acids.

Incorporating Brain-Boosting Foods into the Atkins Diet

Crafting an Atkins Diet that specifically prioritizes cognitive health involves strategic food choices. Women over 60 can customize their dietary approach to include brain-boosting foods that align with the principles of the Atkins Diet. Here are some key considerations:

1. **Fatty Fish:** Integrate fatty fish, such as salmon and mackerel, into the diet to benefit from omega-3 fatty acids. These can be grilled, baked, or incorporated into salads for a brain-boosting meal.

2. **Leafy Greens:** Emphasize low-carb, antioxidant-rich vegetables like spinach, kale, and Swiss chard. These can be incorporated into salads, sautéed as side dishes, or blended into smoothies for a nutrient-packed boost.

3. **Nuts and Seeds:** Include nuts and seeds, such as walnuts, chia seeds, and flaxseeds, as sources of healthy fats and antioxidants. These can be sprinkled on salads, yogurt, or enjoyed as snacks.

4. **Avocados:** Harness the brain-protective power of avocados by incorporating them into meals. Avocados can be sliced onto salads, mashed as a topping, or blended into smoothies for a creamy and nutritious addition.

5. **Olive Oil:** Choose extra virgin olive oil as a primary cooking and dressing oil. Its monounsaturated fats and antioxidant properties contribute to brain health while aligning with the principles of the Atkins Diet.

6. **Berries in Moderation:** While berries are relatively low in carbs, they should be consumed in moderation due to their natural sugars. Berries, such as blueberries and raspberries, can be enjoyed as a flavorful and antioxidant-rich treat.

Practical Strategies for Cognitive Health on the Atkins Diet

Beyond specific food choices, adopting practical strategies can further enhance cognitive health within the framework of the Atkins Diet. Women over 60 can incorporate these strategies into their daily lives to support mental clarity and cognitive function:

1. **Stay Hydrated:** Dehydration can impair cognitive function, so maintaining adequate hydration is crucial. Aim to drink water consistently throughout the day.

2. **Regular Physical Activity:** Engage in regular physical activity, as exercise has been linked to improved cognitive function. Activities like walking, swimming, or yoga can contribute to overall well-being.

3. **Adequate Sleep:** Prioritize sufficient and restful sleep, as inadequate sleep can negatively impact cognitive performance. Establishing a consistent sleep routine and creating a comfortable sleep environment are essential.

4. **Mindful Eating:** Practice mindful eating to cultivate awareness and enjoyment of food. This approach encourages savoring each bite, paying attention to hunger and fullness cues, and fostering a positive relationship with food.

5. **Mental Stimulation:** Challenge the brain with activities that stimulate cognitive function. This can

include reading, puzzles, learning new skills, or engaging in activities that promote mental agility.

6. **Social Connections:** Maintain social connections and engage in meaningful interactions. Social engagement has been associated with cognitive health and emotional well-being.

7. **Stress Management:** Adopt effective stress management techniques, such as meditation, deep breathing, or hobbies, to mitigate the impact of chronic stress on cognitive function.

Personalized Approaches to Cognitive Optimization

Recognizing that each woman over 60 is unique, the Atkins Diet allows for personalized approaches to cognitive optimization. Some individuals may find benefits in incorporating intermittent fasting, which has been linked to cognitive improvements and metabolic benefits. Others may explore specific supplements, guided by healthcare professionals, to address individual nutrient needs for optimal cognitive health.

Additionally, the Atkins Diet can be seamlessly integrated into broader lifestyle practices that prioritize cognitive well-being. Mindfulness practices, such as meditation or yoga, complement the dietary approach by addressing stress and promoting mental clarity.

It's essential for women over 60 to view cognitive health as a holistic endeavor that encompasses nutrition, lifestyle, and personalized strategies. By adopting the Atkins Diet with a focus on cognitive optimization, women can navigate the aging process with resilience, enjoying not only physical vitality but also the richness of mental clarity and cognitive vitality.

Celebrating Cognitive Vitality as a Key Element of Holistic Health

In conclusion, the Atkins Diet, renowned for its impact on weight management and metabolic health, extends its benefits to the realm of cognitive vitality for women over 60. By prioritizing brain-friendly nutrients, supporting blood sugar stability, and leveraging the unique metabolic state of ketosis, the Atkins Diet becomes a powerful ally in the quest for mental clarity.

As women embrace the holistic approach of the Atkins Diet, they not only witness transformations on the scale but also experience the vibrant synergy between mind and body. The journey to holistic health becomes a celebration of cognitive vitality, where mental clarity, focus, and cognitive function are cherished elements of a life lived with purpose and resilience.

In this chapter, women over 60 discover that the Atkins Diet is not merely a dietary plan; it's an invitation to a lifestyle that prioritizes their overall well-being. It's an acknowledgment that health is multifaceted, and cognitive health is a valuable aspect that deserves attention, care, and celebration. By weaving cognitive vitality into the fabric of holistic health, women over 60 can navigate the aging process with grace, wisdom, and the enduring glow of mental clarity.

Embracing Sustainable Lifestyle Changes for Long-Term Success

As women enter the golden years, the pursuit of health extends beyond the conventional focus on weight management. The holistic approach to well-being becomes paramount, encompassing physical, mental, and emotional dimensions. Embracing sustainable lifestyle changes becomes the foundation for long-term success, fostering a balanced and fulfilling life for women over 60.

The Pitfalls of Short-Term Solutions

In the quest for health, many individuals are tempted by short-term solutions promising rapid results. Crash diets, extreme fitness regimens, or other quick fixes may yield temporary changes, but they often lack the sustainability required for long-term success, especially for women over 60.

Short-term solutions can lead to a cycle of yo-yo dieting, where weight is lost and regained, creating frustration and potential health risks. These approaches may overlook the crucial elements of holistic health, neglecting mental and emotional well-being in the pursuit of immediate physical changes. Women over 60, seeking enduring well-being, benefit more from sustainable lifestyle changes that address the broader spectrum of health.

Building Foundations: Sustainable Dietary Choices

The cornerstone of holistic health is sustainable dietary choices that nourish the body and support overall well-being. For women over 60, adopting a sustainable dietary approach involves more than restrictive eating; it's about cultivating a positive relationship with food and making choices that are both nourishing and enjoyable.

1. **Whole, Nutrient-Dense Foods:** Prioritize whole, nutrient-dense foods that provide essential vitamins, minerals, and antioxidants. Incorporate a variety of fruits, vegetables, lean proteins, and healthy fats into meals to ensure a well-rounded and nourishing diet.

2. **Balanced Macronutrients:** Embrace a balanced distribution of macronutrients, including proteins, fats, and carbohydrates. Avoid extreme diets that eliminate entire food groups, as balance is key to sustained energy, satiety, and overall health.

3. **Mindful Eating:** Cultivate mindful eating habits, savoring each bite and paying attention to hunger and fullness cues. Mindful eating fosters a positive relationship with food, promoting a healthier approach to sustenance.

4. **Hydration:** Prioritize hydration by consuming an adequate amount of water throughout the day. Staying well-hydrated supports various bodily functions and contributes to overall vitality.

5. **Flexibility and Moderation:** Embrace flexibility and moderation in dietary choices. Occasional indulgences or deviations from the routine are natural and can be accommodated within a sustainable lifestyle.

Unlocking The Power of Physical Activity

Physical activity is a vital component of holistic health, providing benefits beyond weight management. For women over 60, incorporating sustainable and enjoyable exercise routines contributes to overall well-being and longevity.

1. **Choose Enjoyable Activities:** Select physical activities that bring joy and satisfaction. Whether it's brisk walks, dancing, swimming, or yoga, finding activities that resonate with personal preferences increases the likelihood of long-term adherence.

2. **Consistency Over Intensity:** Prioritize consistency over intensity. Sustainable lifestyle changes in physical activity involve regular, moderate exercise rather than sporadic, intense workouts. Consistency builds endurance and supports lasting health benefits.

3. **Functional Fitness:** Focus on functional fitness that enhances daily life. Strength training, balance exercises, and flexibility routines contribute to improved mobility and independence, aligning with the evolving needs of women over 60.

4. **Adapt to Individual Capabilities:** Acknowledge and adapt to individual capabilities and constraints. Tailor exercise routines to accommodate any pre-existing health conditions, ensuring that physical activity remains a positive and safe experience.

5. **Social Engagement:** Incorporate social elements into physical activity. Joining group classes, walking clubs, or engaging in activities with friends enhances motivation and creates a supportive community around sustainable lifestyle changes.

Prioritizing Mental and Emotional Well-Being

Holistic health for women over 60 extends beyond the physical realm, encompassing mental and emotional well-being. Embracing sustainable lifestyle changes involves nurturing a positive mindset and addressing the emotional aspects of health.

1. **Stress Management:** Prioritize stress management techniques, such as meditation, deep breathing, or mindfulness practices. Chronic stress can impact overall health, and adopting strategies to manage stress contributes to long-term well-being.

2. **Quality Sleep:** Cultivate healthy sleep habits for optimal mental and emotional health. A consistent sleep routine, creating a comfortable sleep environment, and prioritizing sufficient sleep duration are integral to sustainable lifestyle changes.

3. **Cultivate Emotional Resilience:** Build emotional resilience by cultivating a positive mindset and adopting coping strategies for life's challenges. Accepting that setbacks are a natural part of the journey contributes to sustained well-being.

4. **Social Connections:** Foster and maintain social connections. Meaningful relationships and a supportive social network provide emotional nourishment, contributing to a sense of belonging and fulfillment.

5. **Mind-Body Practices:** Explore mind-body practices like yoga or tai chi that integrate physical activity with mental and emotional well-being. These practices offer a holistic approach to health, aligning with sustainable lifestyle changes.

Creating A Supportive Environment

Sustainable lifestyle changes are greatly influenced by the environment in which they occur. Women over 60 can enhance their success by creating a supportive and encouraging environment that aligns with their health goals.

1. **Healthy Home Environment:** Foster a healthy home environment by keeping nutritious foods accessible, creating spaces for physical activity, and promoting a positive atmosphere that encourages well-being.

2. **Communication and Accountability:** Communicate health goals with family or friends and involve them in the journey. Shared goals create accountability and support, making sustainable lifestyle changes a collective effort.

3. **Educational Resources:** Stay informed and access educational resources that align with holistic health goals. Understanding the principles behind sustainable lifestyle changes empowers women over 60 to make informed decisions.

4. **Professional Guidance:** Seek guidance from healthcare professionals, nutritionists, or fitness experts. Tailoring lifestyle changes to individual health needs ensures that choices are sustainable, safe, and optimized for success.

5. **Celebrate Milestones:** Acknowledge and celebrate milestones along the journey. Whether it's achieving a fitness goal, maintaining a balanced diet, or improving emotional well-being, celebrating successes reinforces the sustainability of lifestyle changes.

The Importance of Adaptability

As women over 60 embrace sustainable lifestyle changes, recognizing the importance of adaptability becomes crucial. Life is dynamic, and health goals may evolve based on changing circumstances, preferences, or health conditions. Sustainable lifestyle changes involve a continuous process of assessment, adaptation, and commitment to overall well-being.

1. **Regular Self-Assessment:** Engage in regular self-assessment of health goals, adjusting them based on changing needs or circumstances. Flexibility and adaptability are integral components of sustained well-being.

2. **Reevaluation of Goals:** Periodically reevaluate health goals to ensure they align with personal values and priorities. Adjusting goals allows for continued motivation and commitment to sustainable lifestyle changes.

3. **Open Communication:** Maintain open communication with healthcare professionals or wellness experts. Sharing changes in health status or lifestyle preferences ensures that guidance remains tailored and relevant.

4. **Lifelong Learning:** Embrace a mindset of lifelong learning about health and well-being. Staying informed about new research, trends, and best practices contributes to the ongoing success of sustainable lifestyle changes.

5. **Balancing Enjoyment and Health:** Strive to find the balance between enjoying life and maintaining health. Sustainable lifestyle changes should enhance

the quality of life, allowing women over 60 to relish the journey towards holistic well-being.

The chapter on embracing sustainable lifestyle changes for women over 60 is an invitation to embark on a journey of holistic well-being. Beyond the scale, beyond fleeting solutions, the emphasis is on cultivating enduring health that encompasses the body, mind, and spirit.

By building sustainable foundations through nourishing dietary choices, enjoyable physical activity, and prioritizing mental and emotional well-being, women over 60 set the stage for long-term success. The journey is not about perfection but about progress, adaptability, and a commitment to a life filled with vitality and fulfillment.

As women navigate the path of sustainable lifestyle changes, they discover that each positive choice contributes to a tapestry of well-being. The chapter becomes a guide, a companion, and an affirmation that the pursuit of health is a dynamic and lifelong journey. It is a celebration of the profound impact that sustainable choices can have on the lives of women over 60, fostering not only longevity but a flourishing and purposeful existence.

A Comprehensive Look at The Overall Health Benefits of Atkins

As women navigate the vibrant tapestry of life beyond 60, holistic health becomes a beacon guiding them toward enduring well-being. The Atkins Diet, renowned for its impact on weight management, unveils a comprehensive array of health benefits that extend far beyond the numbers on the scale. In this exploration, we delve into a comprehensive look at how Atkins contributes to the overall health of women in the golden years.

Balancing Blood Sugar Levels: A Foundation for Health

One of the cornerstones of the Atkins Diet is its ability to balance blood sugar levels. For women over 60, this holds profound implications for overall health. The diet's emphasis on reducing the intake of high-glycemic carbohydrates helps prevent rapid spikes and crashes in blood sugar, fostering stability that contributes to sustained energy levels and a reduced risk of insulin resistance.

Stable blood sugar levels are not only crucial for diabetes prevention and management but also play a pivotal role in energy regulation, mood stability, and cognitive function. By curbing the consumption of foods that lead to pronounced blood sugar fluctuations, Atkins becomes a foundational ally in promoting holistic health for women over 60.

Weight Management and Beyond: The Role of Atkins in Body Composition

While weight management is a primary focus of the Atkins Diet, its impact goes beyond the number on the scale. The diet's low-carbohydrate approach encourages the body to utilize stored fat for energy, contributing to more effective weight loss and the preservation of lean muscle mass.

Maintaining muscle mass is particularly significant for women over 60. Beyond aesthetics, lean muscle plays a crucial role in metabolic health, bone density, and functional fitness. The Atkins Diet, by prioritizing protein intake and promoting fat utilization, supports women in achieving and maintaining a healthy body composition that aligns with overall well-being.

Metabolic Magic: Unleashing the Power of Ketosis

At the heart of the Atkins approach is the induction of ketosis, a metabolic state where the body transitions from burning glucose to utilizing ketones derived from fats. While often associated with weight loss, ketosis unveils a realm of health benefits that extend to various facets of well-being for women over 60.

1. **Enhanced Fat Burning:** In ketosis, the body becomes proficient at burning stored fat for energy. This not only aids in weight management but also contributes to improved metabolic health and the reduction of excess body fat, a factor linked to various health risks.

2. **Stable Energy Levels:** The consistent supply of energy from fat metabolism in ketosis results in stable energy levels. For women over 60, this translates to sustained vitality throughout the day, reducing the likelihood of energy crashes and fatigue.

3. **Cognitive Benefits:** Ketones produced during ketosis have been associated with cognitive benefits. Improved mental clarity, focus, and memory are among the cognitive advantages that contribute to overall brain health for women navigating the complexities of aging.

4. **Appetite Regulation:** Ketosis has an appetite-suppressing effect, making it easier for women over 60 to manage portion control and reduce cravings. This contributes to the sustainable nature of the Atkins Diet and supports long-term adherence to healthy eating habits.

Heart Health: Nurturing Cardiovascular Well-Being

Concerns about heart health often intensify with age, making it imperative for women over 60 to adopt dietary practices that promote cardiovascular well-being. The Atkins Diet, when implemented with a focus on high-quality fats and nutrient-dense foods, offers a holistic approach to heart health.

1. **Cholesterol Management:** Contrary to misconceptions, research suggests that the Atkins Diet can positively impact cholesterol levels. The diet has been associated with an increase in "good" HDL cholesterol and improvements in the overall cholesterol profile, addressing a critical aspect of heart health.

2. **Blood Pressure Regulation:** The reduction of refined carbohydrates and sugars in the Atkins Diet may contribute to blood pressure regulation. Maintaining optimal blood pressure levels is essential for cardiovascular health, reducing the risk of heart disease and related complications.

3. **Inflammation Reduction:** Chronic inflammation is a contributing factor to heart disease. The Atkins Diet, with its emphasis on whole, anti-inflammatory foods, offers a dietary approach that supports inflammation reduction, fostering a heart-healthy environment for women over 60.

Bone Health: Strengthening the Foundation

As women age, maintaining strong and healthy bones becomes paramount. The Atkins Diet, through its emphasis on nutrient-dense foods, provides essential vitamins and minerals that contribute to bone health.

1. **Calcium and Vitamin D Intake:** Adequate calcium and vitamin D are vital for bone health. The Atkins Diet encourages the consumption of dairy products, leafy greens, and other sources rich in these nutrients, supporting bone density and strength.

2. **Protein's Role in Bone Health:** Protein, a key component of the Atkins Diet, plays a role in bone health by contributing to the formation and maintenance of bone tissue. For women over 60, preserving bone density is essential in mitigating the risk of osteoporosis and fractures.

3. **Alkaline Diet Benefits:** The low-carbohydrate nature of the Atkins Diet tends to create an alkaline environment in the body. Alkaline diets have been associated with potential benefits for bone health by reducing the loss of calcium from bones.

Gut Health: Nurturing a Flourishing Microbiome

The health of the gut microbiome holds profound implications for overall well-being, influencing digestion, immune function, and even mental health. The Atkins Diet, with its focus on whole foods and limited processed carbohydrates, contributes to a gut-friendly dietary approach for women over 60.

1. **Fiber and Prebiotics:** While the Atkins Diet restricts certain high-carb foods, it encourages the consumption of fiber-rich vegetables and prebiotics. These components support gut health by providing nourishment for beneficial gut bacteria, promoting a diverse and flourishing microbiome.

2. **Reduced Inflammatory Foods:** The limited intake of processed carbohydrates and sugars in the Atkins Diet may contribute to a reduction in inflammatory foods that can negatively impact gut health. By avoiding substances that may irritate the gut lining, women over 60 can foster a digestive environment conducive to well-being.

3. **Balanced Gut Microbiota:** The balance of gut microbiota is essential for immune function and overall health. The Atkins Diet, with its focus on a balanced intake of macronutrients and whole foods, supports a diverse and balanced gut microbiota, contributing to optimal digestive health.

Maintaining Hormonal Harmony: A Menopause-Friendly Approach

For women over 60, navigating the terrain of hormonal changes, particularly during menopause, requires dietary practices that support hormonal balance. The Atkins Diet, with its emphasis on whole foods and balanced macronutrients, offers a menopause-friendly approach.

1. **Protein for Muscle Mass:** Maintaining lean muscle mass becomes crucial during and after menopause. The protein-centric approach of the Atkins Diet supports muscle preservation, helping women over

60 manage changes in metabolism and hormonal fluctuations.

2. **Healthy Fats for Hormones:** Hormones, including those involved in menopause, rely on healthy fats for synthesis. The inclusion of fats like avocados, olive oil, and fatty fish in the Atkins Diet provides essential building blocks for hormonal health.

3. **Blood Sugar Stability:** Menopausal women often experience fluctuations in blood sugar levels. The blood sugar-stabilizing effects of the Atkins Diet can help manage mood swings, energy crashes, and other symptoms associated with hormonal changes.

Enhanced Energy Levels: A Vital Component of Vitality

Energy is the currency of life, and for women over 60, maintaining vibrant energy levels is essential for an active and fulfilling lifestyle. The Atkins Diet, with its unique metabolic effects, contributes to sustained energy throughout the day.

1. **Steady Energy from Fats:** By relying on fats as a primary energy source, the Atkins Diet provides a steady and sustained supply of energy. This contrasts with the energy spikes and crashes associated with high-carbohydrate diets, offering women over 60 a more stable and enduring vitality.

2. **Mitigating Fatigue:** The avoidance of refined carbohydrates and sugars in the Atkins Diet can help mitigate fatigue by preventing rapid fluctuations in blood sugar levels. This is particularly beneficial for women seeking consistent energy to engage in daily activities and pursuits.

3. **Support for Mitochondrial Function:** Mitochondria, the energy-producing powerhouses within cells,

benefit from the metabolic flexibility induced by the Atkins Diet. This support for mitochondrial function contributes to enhanced energy production, vital for overall vitality.

The Atkins Diet emerges as a comprehensive and holistic approach to well-being for women over 60. Beyond its celebrated role in weight management, Atkins unfolds a tapestry of health benefits that touch on various aspects of overall wellness.

By balancing blood sugar levels, optimizing body composition, harnessing the power of ketosis, nurturing heart and bone health, supporting gut microbiota, managing hormonal changes, and enhancing energy levels, the Atkins Diet becomes a multifaceted ally in the pursuit of holistic health.

As women over 60 embark on this journey beyond the scale, they discover that the Atkins Diet is not merely a dietary plan; it's a lifestyle that nurtures and celebrates the richness of life. It is an affirmation that well-being is multifaceted, dynamic, and deeply interconnected. Through the lens of Atkins, women over 60 embrace a holistic approach to health, savoring the vitality, resilience, and fulfillment that accompanies the tapestry of overall wellness.

CHAPTER SEVEN
TAILORING ATKINS TO YOUR TASTE: CUSTOMIZABLE PLANS

Personalizing Your Atkins Journey for Maximum Results

The Atkins Diet, renowned for its effectiveness in weight management and overall health, recognizes that every individual is unique. As women embark on their Atkins journey, the ability to tailor the approach to personal preferences, tastes, and lifestyle becomes a powerful tool for maximizing results. In this chapter, we delve into the art of personalization, exploring how women over 60 can customize their Atkins experience for a truly individualized and effective wellness journey.

Understanding Your Preferences: The Foundation of Personalization

Before delving into the specifics of tailoring Atkins, it's crucial to understand individual preferences. Preferences encompass not only taste but also lifestyle factors, dietary restrictions, and personal goals. Recognizing that every woman over 60 brings a unique set of preferences to the table lays the foundation for a personalized Atkins journey.

1. **Taste Preferences:** Consider the flavors, textures, and types of foods that resonate with you. Whether you lean towards savory or sweet, enjoy rich and hearty meals or prefer lighter options, understanding your taste preferences allows you to create a personalized Atkins plan that aligns with your culinary inclinations.

2. **Dietary Restrictions:** Take note of any dietary restrictions or preferences, such as vegetarianism, gluten intolerance, or specific food allergies. The flexibility of Atkins allows for adaptation to various dietary needs, ensuring that your personalized plan is not only effective but also enjoyable and sustainable.

3. **Lifestyle Considerations:** Factor in your lifestyle, including daily routines, work commitments, and social activities. A personalized Atkins plan integrates seamlessly into your life, making it feasible and realistic to adhere to your chosen dietary approach without feeling restricted or overwhelmed.

4. **Health and Fitness Goals:** Clarify your health and fitness goals, whether they involve weight management, improving energy levels, enhancing mental clarity, or addressing specific health concerns. Tailoring Atkins to your goals ensures that your journey is purposeful and aligned with your vision of overall well-being.

Building your Customized Atkins Plan: A Step-By-Step Guide

Once you've gained insights into your preferences and goals, the next step is to build a customized Atkins plan that maximizes results while catering to your unique needs. This process involves thoughtful consideration of various elements that contribute to a successful and personalized journey.

1. **Choosing Your Carbohydrate Level:** One of the distinctive features of Atkins is its flexibility in carbohydrate intake. Personalizing your Atkins plan begins with choosing the appropriate carbohydrate level based on your goals and preferences.

   - **Induction Phase:** If you're looking for rapid weight loss and metabolic kickstart, the Induction Phase, with its very low-carb approach, may be suitable. This phase typically lasts for a few weeks and involves consuming 20-25 grams of net carbs per day.

   - **Balancing Phase:** For ongoing weight loss or weight maintenance, the Balancing Phase offers a moderate approach, allowing for a gradual increase in carb intake. This phase enables personalization by providing a range of daily net carbs (typically 25-50 grams) based on individual tolerance and goals.

   - **Pre-Maintenance and Maintenance:** As you approach your goal weight, the Pre-Maintenance and Maintenance phases introduce additional flexibility, allowing for a higher carb intake. Personalizing this aspect involves finding the carb level that supports weight maintenance while accommodating individual preferences.

2. **Selecting Protein Sources:** Personalization extends to the selection of protein sources based on taste preferences, dietary choices, and health considerations. Whether you favor animal proteins, plant-based options, or a combination of both, the Atkins Diet provides the flexibility to customize your protein sources.

   - **Animal Proteins:** Options like lean meats, poultry, fish, and eggs are staples in many Atkins plans, offering high-quality protein and essential nutrients. Personalize your protein choices by incorporating your favorite animal-based sources into meals.

   - **Plant-Based Proteins:** For those with vegetarian or plant-based preferences, Atkins accommodates a variety of plant-based protein sources, including tofu, tempeh, legumes, and plant-based protein powders. This allows women over 60 to personalize their Atkins plan while aligning with their dietary choices.

   - **Combining Proteins:** Personalization may involve a combination of animal and plant-based proteins, creating a diverse and satisfying menu. This approach caters to individual tastes while ensuring an adequate intake of essential amino acids.

3. **Embracing Healthy Fats:** The Atkins Diet places a significant emphasis on healthy fats, recognizing their

role in energy, satiety, and overall well-being. Personalizing your fat choices involves selecting options that not only align with your taste preferences but also contribute to your health goals.

- **Avocados and Nuts:** For a creamy and nutrient-dense boost, avocados and nuts offer healthy fats and a satisfying texture. Personalize your Atkins plan by incorporating these options into salads, snacks, or even smoothies.

- **Olive Oil and Fatty Fish:** Choosing heart-healthy fats like olive oil and incorporating fatty fish such as salmon into your meals supports overall cardiovascular health. Personalize your dietary fat sources based on flavor preferences and health considerations.

- **Dairy or Non-Dairy Fats:** Whether you prefer traditional dairy options like butter and cheese or opt for non-dairy alternatives, personalizing your fat sources allows you to create a satisfying and enjoyable eating experience.

4. **Customizing Vegetable Intake:** While vegetables are a key component of the Atkins Diet, personalization comes into play when selecting the types and amounts of vegetables that suit your taste and dietary preferences.

- **Leafy Greens:** If you enjoy the freshness of leafy greens, personalize your Atkins plan by incorporating options like spinach, kale, and arugula into salads, stir-fries, or as side dishes.

- **Colorful Vegetables:** For those who prefer a variety of colors and textures, customize your vegetable intake with an array of bell peppers, tomatoes, carrots, and other colorful options. Personalization ensures a visually appealing and nutrient-rich plate.

- **Cruciferous Vegetables:** Broccoli, cauliflower, Brussels sprouts, and other cruciferous vegetables offer versatility in both flavor and preparation. Personalize your Atkins journey by including these options in roasted dishes, soups, or as standalone sides.

5. **Snacking Strategies:** Personalizing your Atkins plan includes establishing strategies for snacks that align with your preferences and lifestyle. Whether you're a fan of savory or sweet snacks, personalization ensures that your snack choices contribute to your overall well-being.

- **Savory Snacks:** Options like cheese, olives, and sliced vegetables can be personalized to create satisfying and savory snacks. Pairing these with a protein source provides a balanced and flavorful snack option.

- **Sweet Treats:** For those with a sweet tooth, personalization may involve incorporating sugar-free desserts, berries with whipped cream, or dark chocolate into your snack repertoire. These options cater to cravings while adhering to Atkins principles.

- **Timing and Frequency:** Personalize your snacking schedule based on your daily routine and preferences. Whether you prefer multiple small snacks throughout the day or a more structured approach with larger meals, customization ensures that your Atkins plan is tailored to your lifestyle.

Adapting Atkins to Cultural Preferences and Special Occasions

The beauty of the Atkins Diet lies in its adaptability to diverse cultural preferences and special occasions. Women over 60 can personalize their Atkins journey while embracing cultural traditions or enjoying special events without compromising their health goals.

1. **Cultural Preferences:** If cultural or regional cuisines play a significant role in your dietary preferences, personalize your Atkins plan by adapting traditional recipes to align with the principles of the diet. Whether it's incorporating spices, choosing local ingredients, or modifying cooking methods, personalization allows you to enjoy familiar flavors while staying on track.

2. **Social and Family Gatherings:** Special occasions often revolve around shared meals with family and friends. Personalizing your Atkins plan involves navigating social gatherings by making mindful choices that align with your dietary goals. Whether it's choosing protein-rich options, enjoying a variety of vegetables, or indulging in Atkins-friendly desserts, customization ensures that you can participate in festivities without straying from your path.

3. **Traveling on Atkins:** Personalization extends to navigating dietary choices while traveling. Whether exploring new cuisines or adhering to familiar options, women over 60 can customize their Atkins plan to suit travel-related challenges. This may

involve planning ahead, making informed choices at restaurants, and incorporating convenient Atkins-friendly snacks into the travel routine.

Monitoring Progress and Adjusting Personalized Plans

A personalized Atkins journey involves continuous monitoring of progress and making adjustments as needed. Tracking key indicators and being attuned to your body's responses allow women over 60 to refine and optimize their personalized plans for sustained success.

1. **Weight and Body Composition:** Regularly monitoring weight and body composition provides valuable insights into the effectiveness of your personalized Atkins plan. Adjusting carbohydrate levels, protein intake, or overall calorie intake based on progress ensures that your plan remains aligned with your weight management goals.

2. **Energy Levels and Well-Being:** Pay attention to your energy levels, mood, and overall well-being. Personalization may involve tweaking macronutrient ratios, adjusting meal timing, or incorporating specific foods that enhance your vitality and satisfaction with the Atkins lifestyle.

3. **Blood Sugar Levels:** For those with specific health concerns, monitoring blood sugar levels can guide personalization efforts. Adjusting carbohydrate intake, experimenting with meal timing, and incorporating blood sugar-friendly foods contribute to overall health and metabolic stability.

4. **Adapting to Changing Needs:** As women over 60 experience changes in lifestyle, health status, or

preferences, the adaptability of Atkins shines. Personalizing your plan involves adapting to changing needs by modifying carbohydrate levels, adjusting food choices, and incorporating new strategies that align with your evolving journey.

5. **Seeking Professional Guidance:** Consulting with healthcare professionals, nutritionists, or Atkins experts adds an extra layer of personalization. These professionals can provide personalized guidance based on individual health needs, ensuring that your Atkins journey is optimized for maximum results and overall well-being.

Personalizing your Atkins journey as a woman over 60 is a powerful approach to achieving maximum results in weight management, overall health, and well-being. By understanding your preferences, building a customized Atkins plan, adapting to cultural preferences and special occasions, and monitoring progress with a keen eye, you create a tailored path to success.

The art of personalization transforms Atkins from a standardized diet plan into a dynamic and individualized lifestyle. It celebrates the diversity of tastes, preferences, and goals that women over 60 bring to their wellness journey. As you embark on your personalized Atkins adventure, relish the freedom to shape your dietary path, savor the flavors that bring you joy, and celebrate the unique and empowering experience of making Atkins truly your own.

Adapting The Diet to Your Preferences and Lifestyle

As women over 60 embrace the Atkins Diet, the concept of personalization emerges as a guiding principle, offering the freedom to tailor the diet to individual preferences and lifestyles. In this chapter, we explore the art of adapting Atkins to your taste, delving into the myriad ways in which the diet can be personalized to align with unique culinary inclinations, dietary needs, and daily routines. By understanding the nuances of personalization, women over 60 can unlock the full potential of Atkins, making it not just a diet but a personalized journey towards holistic well-being.

The Canvas of Culinary Preferences: Crafting Flavorful Atkins Meals

1. **Flavor Profiles and Culinary Diversity:** Atkins is not a one-size-fits-all approach, and neither should the flavors be. Personalizing your Atkins journey involves embracing a diverse array of flavor profiles that resonate with your culinary preferences. Whether you savor the warmth of spices, the freshness of herbs, or the richness of umami, the diet's flexibility allows for the creation of meals that bring joy to your palate.

   - *Spice Enthusiasts:* For those who appreciate bold and spicy flavors, Atkins offers a canvas to experiment with various spices like cumin, paprika, and chili powder. Spice-infused dishes not only add depth to the taste but also contribute to the metabolic benefits associated with certain spices.

   - *Herb Aficionados:* If the aromatic allure of herbs captivates your senses, personalize your

Atkins meals by incorporating fresh herbs like basil, cilantro, and parsley. Herb-infused dishes not only enhance the flavor but also contribute to the diet's nutrient density.

- **Umami Lovers:** For those drawn to the savory richness of umami, Atkins provides opportunities to explore umami-rich ingredients such as mushrooms, tomatoes, and soy-based products. Crafting meals that satisfy umami cravings ensures that your Atkins experience is both delicious and fulfilling.

2. **Customizing Protein Palates:** Protein is a cornerstone of the Atkins Diet, and personalization extends to the types of protein sources that grace your plate. Tailoring your protein choices ensures that meals are not only nutritionally balanced but also aligned with your taste preferences.

- **Meat Enthusiasts:** If you revel in the savory goodness of meat, personalize your Atkins plan by exploring a variety of meat options, from lean cuts of beef and poultry to succulent lamb or pork. Grilling, roasting, or slow-cooking meats allows for a range of textures and flavors.

- **Seafood Connoisseurs:** Seafood lovers can personalize their Atkins meals with a bounty from the ocean. Salmon, shrimp, tuna, and other seafood options offer a delectable way to incorporate essential omega-3 fatty acids, supporting heart health while indulging in flavors of the sea.

- **Plant-Based Explorers:** For those who prefer plant-based proteins, Atkins is adaptable to a variety of options such as tofu, tempeh, legumes, and plant-based protein sources. Personalizing your protein choices ensures that the diet accommodates diverse dietary preferences.

3. **The Vegetable Mosaic: Crafting Colorful and Nutrient-Rich Meals:** Vegetables play a pivotal role in the Atkins Diet, and personalization involves creating a vibrant vegetable mosaic that not only supports nutritional goals but also appeals to your visual and culinary senses.

   - **Colorful Creations:** Personalize your vegetable intake by embracing a spectrum of colors on your plate. Bell peppers, tomatoes, leafy greens, and vibrant cruciferous vegetables offer a palette that not only enhances nutritional diversity but also adds visual appeal to your meals.

   - **Texture Exploration:** The Atkins Diet allows for creativity in texture, enabling you to personalize meals based on your preference for crunch, tenderness, or a combination of both. Roasting vegetables for a crispy texture or incorporating sautéed greens for tenderness adds a personalized touch to your culinary repertoire.

   - **Seasonal Variations:** Personalization extends to embracing seasonal produce, allowing you to tailor your meals to the offerings of each season. Whether it's hearty root vegetables in the fall or fresh berries in the summer, aligning with seasonal produce ensures variety and freshness in your Atkins journey.

The Lifestyle Connection: Aligning Atkins with Daily Routines

1. **Meal Timing and Frequency:** One of the hallmarks of personalizing Atkins is adapting meal timing and frequency to your lifestyle. Whether you prefer three square meals a day, intermittent fasting, or a more frequent grazing approach, the diet accommodates various meal cadences to suit your daily routine.

   - **_Intermittent Fasting:_** For those who find benefit in intermittent fasting, Atkins can be personalized to align with fasting windows. Timing meals strategically within the feeding window allows for effective adherence to both Atkins principles and intermittent fasting protocols.

   - **_Structured Meals:_** If structured meals resonate with your routine, personalization involves planning satisfying and nutrient-dense breakfasts, lunches, and dinners. Creating meals that align with your daily rhythm ensures that Atkins seamlessly integrates into your lifestyle.

   - **_Snacking Strategies:_** Personalizing Atkins extends to snacking preferences. Whether you prefer small, frequent snacks throughout the day or structured meals with minimal snacking, adapting the diet to your snacking habits ensures that your energy levels are sustained without compromising your health goals.

2. **On-the-Go Adaptations:** Life is dynamic, and personalizing Atkins involves adapting the diet to on-

the-go scenarios. Whether you're a busy professional, a traveler, or someone with a bustling schedule, tailoring Atkins to your lifestyle ensures that you can maintain your dietary preferences even in the midst of a hectic routine.

- **_Convenient Snacks:_** Atkins offers a range of convenient and portable snacks that cater to various taste preferences. Personalization involves choosing snacks that not only align with the diet's principles but also suit your on-the-go lifestyle, providing a quick and satisfying solution when time is of the essence.

- **_Restaurant Navigation:_** Dining out is a common aspect of social and professional life. Personalizing Atkins includes developing strategies for navigating restaurant menus, making informed choices, and enjoying meals that align with your dietary preferences, even when away from home.

- **_Travel-Friendly Choices:_** For women over 60 who enjoy traveling, personalization involves selecting Atkins-friendly options that are easy to carry and consume while on the move. Incorporating travel-friendly snacks and making smart choices at airports or during road trips ensures that Atkins remains an integral part of your journey.

3. **Culinary Creativity in the Kitchen:** Personalization extends to the kitchen, where culinary creativity flourishes. Whether you're an avid cook or someone who prefers quick and easy recipes, adapting Atkins to your cooking style allows you to enjoy the process

of preparing meals that resonate with your taste buds.

- **Simple and Quick Recipes:** For those with a busy lifestyle, personalization involves exploring simple and quick Atkins recipes that require minimal preparation time. Efficient cooking methods, such as sheet pan dinners or one-pot meals, cater to time constraints without compromising on flavor.

- **Gourmet Exploration:** Culinary enthusiasts can personalize Atkins by embarking on a gourmet exploration of flavors and techniques. Experimenting with herbs, spices, and cooking methods allows for a nuanced and sophisticated Atkins experience that aligns with your culinary passions.

- **Family-Friendly Options:** Personalization involves adapting Atkins to family meals, ensuring that the diet accommodates the preferences of all family members. Crafting family-friendly recipes that are both nutritious and delicious fosters a shared appreciation for the Atkins lifestyle.

Celebrating Special Occasions: Balancing Indulgence and Wellness

1. **Birthday Bashes and Festive Feasts:** Personalizing Atkins involves navigating special occasions and celebrations without compromising health goals. Whether it's a birthday celebration, a holiday feast, or a festive gathering, adapting Atkins to special occasions allows women over 60 to enjoy the festivities while maintaining balance.

   - *Low-Carb Celebrations:* Personalize special occasions by incorporating low-carb versions of favorite dishes. From cauliflower mash to zucchini noodles, Atkins-friendly alternatives allow you to indulge in celebratory meals without deviating from the principles of the diet.

   - *Smart Dessert Choices:* For those with a sweet tooth, personalization involves making smart dessert choices during special occasions. Opting for sugar-free desserts, dark chocolate, or Atkins-approved treats allows for indulgence without compromising on health goals.

   - *Balanced Alcohol Choices:* Celebrations often include toasts and libations. Personalizing Atkins involves making balanced alcohol choices that align with the principles of the diet. Choosing dry wines, spirits with low-carb mixers, or Atkins-friendly cocktails ensures that celebrations are enjoyed without straying from the path of wellness.

2. **Cultural Traditions and Culinary Heritage:** Personalizing Atkins extends to cultural traditions and culinary heritage. Whether you have cultural preferences deeply rooted in your heritage or enjoy exploring diverse cuisines, adapting Atkins to cultural contexts allows for a rich and personalized dietary experience.

   - *Cultural Adaptations:* Personalize Atkins by adapting traditional recipes to align with the diet's principles. Whether it's tweaking ingredients, modifying cooking methods, or incorporating Atkins-friendly alternatives, cultural adaptations ensure that heritage and dietary goals coexist harmoniously.

   - *Exploring Global Cuisines:* For culinary explorers who appreciate global cuisines, personalization involves experimenting with Atkins-friendly versions of dishes from around the world. Embracing the flavors of Mediterranean, Asian, or Latin cuisines allows for a diverse and satisfying Atkins experience.

   - *Seasonal Celebrations:* Cultural traditions often involve seasonal celebrations and festivities. Personalizing Atkins includes crafting meals that resonate with seasonal ingredients and traditional culinary practices, ensuring that cultural celebrations are both meaningful and health conscious.

Continuous Refinement: Listening To Your Body and Evolving Preferences

1. **Attuned Eating and Intuitive Choices:** As women over 60 personalize their Atkins journey, a key aspect involves attuned eating and intuitive choices. Listening to your body's signals, recognizing hunger and satiety cues, and making choices based on intuition contribute to a dynamic and evolving relationship with the diet.

   - *Mindful Eating Practices:* Personalization involves embracing mindful eating practices that enhance the enjoyment and satisfaction derived from meals. Paying attention to flavors, textures, and the overall dining experience fosters a connection between body and mind.

   - *Intuitive Food Selection:* Personalize Atkins by intuitively selecting foods that align with your body's needs and preferences. Whether it's choosing ingredients that provide sustained energy or incorporating foods that contribute to overall well-being, intuitive food selection is a cornerstone of personalization.

   - *Adapting to Changing Preferences:* As preferences evolve with time, personalization involves adapting Atkins to changing taste buds and culinary inclinations. Experimenting with new recipes, exploring different cuisines, and incorporating seasonal variations ensure that the diet remains a dynamic and satisfying journey.

2. **Optimizing for Wellness Goals:** Personalizing Atkins is an ongoing process of optimization, aligning the diet with evolving wellness goals. Whether your focus is on weight management, metabolic health, or overall vitality, refining your Atkins plan to meet specific wellness objectives ensures that the diet remains a powerful tool in achieving optimal health.

   - *Weight Management Adjustments:* For women over 60 focused on weight management, personalization involves making adjustments to carbohydrate levels, protein intake, and overall calorie consumption based on progress and goals. Fine-tuning these elements ensures that Atkins remains an effective strategy for weight-related objectives.

   - *Metabolic Wellness Strategies:* Personalization extends to strategies that support metabolic wellness. Adapting Atkins to incorporate foods and practices that contribute to stable blood sugar levels, enhanced energy metabolism, and overall metabolic health aligns with wellness goals for women over 60.

   - *Comprehensive Well-Being:* Beyond weight and metabolic considerations, personalization involves a holistic approach to well-being. Adapting Atkins to address specific health concerns, enhance mental clarity, or support emotional balance ensures that the diet becomes a personalized roadmap to comprehensive wellness.

Tailoring Atkins to your taste as a woman over 60 is a dynamic and empowering journey. The diet transcends a one-size-fits-all approach, inviting individuals to infuse their unique preferences, culinary passions, and lifestyle nuances into the Atkins canvas. By embracing the art of personalization, women over 60 transform Atkins from a dietary plan into a personalized lifestyle that celebrates the joy of nourishing the body, savoring diverse flavors, and achieving sustainable well-being.

As you navigate the vast landscape of personalization within Atkins, relish the freedom to craft meals that reflect your personality, align with your daily rhythms, and harmonize with your cultural traditions. The journey towards sustainable well-being is not about rigid rules but about the

Atkins For Every Palate: Delicious and Nutrient-Rich Recipes

Embarking on the Atkins journey involves more than just dietary changes; it's an opportunity for culinary exploration and the creation of delicious, nutrient-rich meals. In this chapter, we delve into the world of recipes tailored to suit every palate. Whether you are a fan of savory delights, have a sweet tooth, or savor the diversity of global cuisines, Atkins provides a canvas for crafting meals that are not only satisfying but also contribute to your overall well-being.

1. Savory Delights: Flavorful Meals for every Taste Bud

Atkins offers a plethora of savory recipes that cater to a variety of tastes. From hearty breakfasts to satisfying dinners, these recipes not only align with the principles of the diet but also celebrate the rich tapestry of flavors that women over 60 can savor.

1. Egg and Avocado Breakfast Bowl

Ingredients:

- 2 eggs
- 1 ripe avocado
- Cherry tomatoes, halved
- Fresh cilantro, chopped
- Salt and pepper to taste

Instructions:

1. Poach or fry the eggs to your liking.
2. Cut the avocado in half and remove the pit.
3. Place the poached or fried eggs into the avocado halves.
4. Add halved cherry tomatoes on top.
5. Sprinkle with fresh cilantro, salt, and pepper.

Nutritional Information:

- Calories: 380
- Protein: 13g
- Fat: 32g
- Carbohydrates: 15g
- Fiber: 10g
- Sugar: 2g

2. Grilled Chicken Caesar Salad

Ingredients:

- Grilled chicken breast, sliced
- Romaine lettuce, chopped
- Cherry tomatoes, halved
- Parmesan cheese, shaved
- Caesar dressing (low-carb)

Instructions:

1. Grill the chicken breast until fully cooked, then slice it.
2. In a large bowl, toss together the chopped romaine lettuce and cherry tomatoes.

3. Add the sliced grilled chicken on top.

4. Sprinkle shaved Parmesan cheese over the salad.

5. Drizzle with your favorite low-carb Caesar dressing.

Nutritional Information:

- Calories: 420

- Protein: 35g

- Fat: 26g

- Carbohydrates: 10g

- Fiber: 5g

- Sugar: 3g

3. Zucchini Noodles with Pesto and Cherry Tomatoes

Ingredients:

- Zucchini, spiralized

- Cherry tomatoes, halved

- Pesto sauce (low-carb)

- Olive oil

- Pine nuts (optional)

Instructions:

1. Spiralize the zucchini into noodles.

2. In a pan, sauté the zucchini noodles in olive oil until tender.

3. Toss the zucchini noodles with cherry tomatoes.

4. Drizzle with your favorite low-carb pesto sauce.

5. Optionally, sprinkle with pine nuts for added crunch.

Nutritional Information:

- Calories: 280

- Protein: 6g

- Fat: 23g

- Carbohydrates: 10g

- Fiber: 3g

- Sugar: 5g

4. Avocado Chocolate Mousse

Ingredients:

- Ripe avocados, peeled and pitted

- Unsweetened cocoa powder

- Low-carb sweetener (e.g., Stevia)

- Vanilla extract

- Almond milk

Instructions:

1. In a blender, combine ripe avocados, cocoa powder, sweetener, and a splash of almond milk.

2. Blend until smooth and creamy.

3. Add vanilla extract to taste and blend again.

4. Chill the mousse in the refrigerator before serving.

Nutritional Information:

- Calories: 220

- Protein: 3g

- Fat: 18g

- Carbohydrates: 14g

- Fiber: 8g / Sugar: 1g

5. Berries and Cream Parfait

Ingredients:

- Mixed berries (e.g., strawberries, blueberries, raspberries)
- Heavy cream
- Vanilla extract
- Low-carb sweetener
- Chopped nuts for garnish

Instructions:

1. In a bowl, mix heavy cream with vanilla extract and sweetener to taste.
2. Whip the cream until stiff peaks form.
3. Layer mixed berries and whipped cream in serving glasses.
4. Repeat the layers, ending with a dollop of whipped cream on top.
5. Garnish with chopped nuts for added crunch.

Nutritional Information:

- Calories: 300
- Protein: 3g
- Fat: 28g
- Carbohydrates: 10g
- Fiber: 5g
- Sugar: 3g

6. Coconut Almond Energy Bites

Ingredients:

- Shredded coconut
- Almond flour
- Coconut oil
- Low-carb sweetener
- Almond extract

Instructions:

1. In a bowl, combine shredded coconut, almond flour, melted coconut oil, sweetener, and almond extract.
2. Mix until a dough-like consistency forms.
3. Roll the mixture into small energy bites.
4. Place the energy bites in the refrigerator to set.
5. Enjoy as a sweet and nutty snack.

Nutritional Information:

- Calories: 120
- Protein: 2g
- Fat: 10g
- Carbohydrates: 6g
- Fiber: 3g
- Sugar: 2g

7. Mediterranean Cauliflower Rice Bowl

Ingredients:

- Cauliflower rice
- Grilled chicken or shrimp
- Cherry tomatoes, halved
- Cucumber, diced
- Feta cheese, crumbled
- Kalamata olives
- Tzatziki sauce (low-carb)

Instructions:

1. Prepare cauliflower rice by pulsing cauliflower in a food processor.
2. Grill chicken or shrimp until fully cooked.
3. In a bowl, layer cauliflower rice with grilled protein, cherry tomatoes, cucumber, feta cheese, and Kalamata olives.
4. Drizzle with low-carb tzatziki sauce.

Nutritional Information:

- Calories: 380
- Protein: 25g
- Fat: 20g
- Carbohydrates: 15g
- Fiber: 8g
- Sugar: 6g

8. Spicy Thai Zoodle Stir-Fry

Ingredients:

- Zucchini noodles
- Cooked shrimp or tofu
- Bell peppers, sliced
- Snow peas
- Green onions, chopped
- Thai red curry paste
- Coconut aminos

Instructions:

1. In a wok, stir-fry zucchini noodles, cooked shrimp or tofu, sliced bell peppers, and snow peas.
2. Add Thai red curry paste and coconut aminos to taste.
3. Continue to stir-fry until the vegetables are tender.
4. Garnish with chopped green onions before serving.

Nutritional Information:

- Calories: 320
- Protein: 15g
- Fat: 18g
- Carbohydrates: 12g
- Fiber: 4g
- Sugar: 6g

9. Indian Cauliflower and Chickpea Curry

Ingredients:

- Cauliflower florets
- Chickpeas
- Tomato, diced
- Onion, finely chopped
- Garlic and ginger, minced
- Curry spices (cumin, coriander, turmeric, garam masala)
- Coconut milk (unsweetened)

Instructions:

1. Sauté onions, garlic, and ginger until softened.
2. Add diced tomatoes and spices, cooking until fragrant.
3. Add cauliflower florets and chickpeas, stirring to coat in the spice mixture.
4. Pour in unsweetened coconut milk and simmer until the cauliflower is tender.
5. Serve over cauliflower rice.

Nutritional Information:

- Calories: 340
- Protein: 12g
- Fat: 15g
- Carbohydrates: 18g
- Fiber: 6g
- Sugar: 4g

11. Protein-Packed Breakfast Bowl (Energize Your Morning)

Ingredients:

- 2 eggs
- 1 ripe avocado
- Cherry tomatoes, halved
- Fresh cilantro, chopped
- Salt and pepper to taste

Instructions:

1. Poach or fry the eggs to your liking.
2. Cut the avocado in half and remove the pit.
3. Place the poached or fried eggs into the avocado halves.
4. Add halved cherry tomatoes on top.
5. Sprinkle with fresh cilantro, salt, and pepper.

Nutritional Information:

- Calories: 380
- Protein: 13g
- Fat: 32g
- Carbohydrates: 15g
- Fiber: 10g
- Sugar: 2g

12. Grilled Chicken Caesar Salad (A Classic Reinvented)

Ingredients:

- Grilled chicken breast, sliced
- Romaine lettuce, chopped
- Cherry tomatoes, halved
- Parmesan cheese, shaved
- Caesar dressing (low-carb)

Instructions:

1. Grill the chicken breast until fully cooked, then slice it.
2. In a large bowl, toss together the chopped romaine lettuce and cherry tomatoes.
3. Add the sliced grilled chicken on top.
4. Sprinkle shaved Parmesan cheese over the salad.
5. Drizzle with your favorite low-carb Caesar dressing.

Nutritional Information:

- Calories: 420
- Protein: 35g
- Fat: 26g
- Carbohydrates: 10g
- Fiber: 5g
- Sugar: 3g

13. Zucchini Noodles with Pesto and Cherry Tomatoes (Carb-Conscious Pasta)

Ingredients:

- Zucchini, spiralized
- Cherry tomatoes, halved
- Pesto sauce (low-carb)
- Olive oil
- Pine nuts (optional)

Instructions:

1. Spiralize the zucchini into noodles.
2. In a pan, sauté the zucchini noodles in olive oil until tender.
3. Toss the zucchini noodles with cherry tomatoes.
4. Drizzle with your favorite low-carb pesto sauce.
5. Optionally, sprinkle with pine nuts for added crunch.

Nutritional Information:

- Calories: 280
- Protein: 6g
- Fat: 23g
- Carbohydrates: 10g
- Fiber: 3g
- Sugar: 5g

14. Avocado Chocolate Mousse (Decadent and Wholesome)

Ingredients:

- Ripe avocados, peeled and pitted
- Unsweetened cocoa powder
- Low-carb sweetener (e.g., Stevia)
- Vanilla extract
- Almond milk

Instructions:

1. In a blender, combine ripe avocados, cocoa powder, sweetener, and a splash of almond milk.
2. Blend until smooth and creamy.
3. Add vanilla extract to taste and blend again.
4. Chill the mousse in the refrigerator before serving.

Nutritional Information:

- Calories: 220
- Protein: 3g
- Fat: 18g
- Carbohydrates: 14g
- Fiber: 8g
- Sugar: 1g

15. Berries and Cream Parfait (Sweet Delight without Guilt)

Ingredients:

- Mixed berries (e.g., strawberries, blueberries, raspberries)
- Heavy cream
- Vanilla extract
- Low-carb sweetener
- Chopped nuts for garnish

Instructions:

1. In a bowl, mix heavy cream with vanilla extract and sweetener to taste.
2. Whip the cream until stiff peaks form.
3. Layer mixed berries and whipped cream in serving glasses.
4. Repeat the layers, ending with a dollop of whipped cream on top.
5. Garnish with chopped nuts for added crunch.

Nutritional Information:

- Calories: 300
- Protein: 3g
- Fat: 28g
- Carbohydrates: 10g
- Fiber: 5g
- Sugar: 3g

16. Coconut Almond Energy Bites (Snack Smart and Satisfying)

Ingredients:

- Shredded coconut
- Almond flour
- Coconut oil
- Low-carb sweetener
- Almond extract

Instructions:

1. In a bowl, combine shredded coconut, almond flour, melted coconut oil, sweetener, and almond extract.
2. Mix until a dough-like consistency forms.
3. Roll the mixture into small energy bites.
4. Place the energy bites in the refrigerator to set.
5. Enjoy as a sweet and nutty snack.

Nutritional Information:

- Calories: 120
- Protein: 2g
- Fat: 10g
- Carbohydrates: 6g
- Fiber: 3g
- Sugar: 2g

17. Mediterranean Cauliflower Rice Bowl (A Flavorful Escape)

Ingredients:

- Cauliflower rice
- Grilled chicken or shrimp
- Cherry tomatoes, halved
- Cucumber, diced
- Feta cheese, crumbled
- Kalamata olives
- Tzatziki sauce (low-carb)

Instructions:

1. Prepare cauliflower rice by pulsing cauliflower in a food processor.
2. Grill chicken or shrimp until fully cooked.
3. In a bowl, layer cauliflower rice with grilled protein, cherry tomatoes, cucumber, feta cheese, and Kalamata olives.
4. Drizzle with low-carb tzatziki sauce.

Nutritional Information:

- Calories: 380
- Protein: 25g
- Fat: 20g
- Carbohydrates: 15g
- Fiber: 8g
- Sugar: 6g

18. Grilled Salmon with Lemon-Dill Sauce (Omega-3 Boost)

Ingredients:

- 4 salmon fillets
- 2 tablespoons olive oil
- Salt and pepper to taste
- Fresh dill, chopped
- 1 lemon (zested and juiced)

Instructions:

1. Preheat the grill to medium-high heat.
2. Rub salmon fillets with olive oil and season with salt and pepper.
3. Grill salmon for 4-5 minutes per side or until cooked through.
4. In a small bowl, mix chopped dill, lemon zest, and lemon juice.
5. Drizzle the lemon-dill sauce over grilled salmon before serving.

Nutritional Information:

- Calories: 350
- Protein: 30g
- Fat: 22g
- Carbohydrates: 1g
- Fiber: 0g
- Sugar: 0g

19. Cauliflower and Broccoli Alfredo Bake (Low-Carb Comfort)

Ingredients:

- 1 cauliflower head, cut into florets
- 2 cups broccoli florets
- 1 cup heavy cream
- 1 cup grated Parmesan cheese
- 2 cloves garlic, minced
- Salt and pepper to taste

Instructions:

1. Preheat the oven to 375°F (190°C).
2. Steam cauliflower and broccoli until tender-crisp.
3. In a saucepan, heat heavy cream, Parmesan cheese, minced garlic, salt, and pepper until cheese is melted.
4. Combine steamed vegetables with Alfredo sauce and transfer to a baking dish.
5. Bake for 20-25 minutes or until bubbly and golden.

Nutritional Information:

- Calories: 280
- Protein: 12g
- Fat: 20g
- Carbohydrates: 10g
- Fiber: 4g
- Sugar: 3g

20. Spinach and Feta Stuffed Chicken Breast (Mediterranean Delight)

Ingredients:

- 4 boneless, skinless chicken breasts
- 2 cups fresh spinach, chopped
- 1/2 cup feta cheese, crumbled
- 1 tablespoon olive oil
- 1 teaspoon dried oregano
- Salt and pepper to taste

Instructions:

1. Preheat the oven to 400°F (200°C).
2. In a skillet, sauté chopped spinach in olive oil until wilted.
3. Mix sautéed spinach with crumbled feta, dried oregano, salt, and pepper.
4. Cut a pocket into each chicken breast and stuff with the spinach and feta mixture.
5. Bake for 25-30 minutes or until chicken is cooked through.

Nutritional Information:

- Calories: 320
- Protein: 35g
- Fat: 15g
- Carbohydrates: 4g
- Fiber: 2g / Sugar: 1g

21. Eggplant Lasagna with Ground Turkey (Low-Carb Italian Feast)

Ingredients:

- 1 large eggplant, sliced
- 1 pound ground turkey
- 1 cup ricotta cheese
- 1 cup marinara sauce (sugar-free)
- 1 cup mozzarella cheese, shredded
- Italian seasoning, to taste

Instructions:

1. Preheat the oven to 375°F (190°C).
2. Grill or roast eggplant slices until tender.
3. In a skillet, brown ground turkey and season with Italian seasoning.
4. In a baking dish, layer grilled eggplant, ground turkey, ricotta cheese, marinara sauce, and mozzarella.
5. Repeat layers and bake for 25-30 minutes.

Nutritional Information:

- Calories: 380
- Protein: 28g
- Fat: 22g
- Carbohydrates: 10g
- Fiber: 4g
- Sugar: 5g

22. Shrimp and Avocado Salad (Fresh and Flavorful)

Ingredients:

- 1 pound shrimp, peeled and deveined
- 2 avocados, diced
- Cherry tomatoes, halved
- Red onion, finely chopped
- Fresh cilantro, chopped
- Lime vinaigrette (lime juice, olive oil, salt, pepper)

Instructions:

1. Grill or sauté shrimp until pink and opaque.
2. In a bowl, combine diced avocados, cherry tomatoes, chopped red onion, and grilled shrimp.
3. In a separate bowl, whisk together lime juice, olive oil, salt, and pepper to make the vinaigrette.
4. Drizzle the vinaigrette over the salad and toss gently.

Nutritional Information:

- Calories: 310
- Protein: 25g
- Fat: 20g
- Carbohydrates: 12g
- Fiber: 7g
- Sugar: 2g

23. Turkey and Vegetable Stir-Fry (Quick and Nutrient-Packed)

Ingredients:

- 1 pound turkey breast, thinly sliced
- Broccoli florets
- Bell peppers, sliced
- Snap peas
- Ginger and garlic, minced
- Soy sauce (low-sodium)

Instructions:

1. In a wok or skillet, stir-fry sliced turkey until browned and cooked through.
2. Add broccoli, bell peppers, snap peas, ginger, and garlic to the wok.
3. Continue stir-frying until vegetables are tender-crisp.
4. Drizzle with low-sodium soy sauce and toss to coat.

Nutritional Information:

- Calories: 290
- Protein: 30g
- Fat: 8g
- Carbohydrates: 14g
- Fiber: 5g
- Sugar: 4g

24. Blueberry and Almond Chia Pudding (Sweet Indulgence, Low-Carb Style)

Ingredients:

- 1/4 cup chia seeds
- 1 cup unsweetened almond milk
- Blueberries
- Almonds, sliced
- Vanilla extract
- Low-carb sweetener

Instructions:

1. In a jar, mix chia seeds with almond milk, vanilla extract, and sweetener.
2. Stir well and refrigerate for at least 4 hours or overnight.
3. Layer chia pudding with fresh blueberries and sliced almonds before serving.

Nutritional Information:

- Calories: 220
- Protein: 8g
- Fat: 16g
- Carbohydrates: 15g
- Fiber: 9g
- Sugar: 3g

25. Quinoa and Vegetable Stuffed Bell Peppers (Plant-Powered Protein)

Ingredients:

- 4 bell peppers, halved
- 1 cup quinoa, cooked
- Mixed vegetables (zucchini, cherry tomatoes, spinach)
- Feta cheese, crumbled
- Olive oil
- Italian seasoning
- Salt and pepper to taste

Instructions:

1. Preheat the oven to 375°F (190°C).
2. In a bowl, mix cooked quinoa with chopped vegetables and feta cheese.
3. Drizzle olive oil and season with Italian seasoning, salt, and pepper.
4. Stuff the bell peppers with the quinoa mixture.
5. Bake for 25-30 minutes or until peppers are tender.

Nutritional Information:

- Calories: 320
- Protein: 12g
- Fat: 10g
- Carbohydrates: 45g
- Fiber: 8g / Sugar: 4g

26. Salmon and Asparagus Foil Packets (Omega-3 Powerhouse)

Ingredients:

- 4 salmon fillets
- Asparagus spears
- Lemon slices
- Garlic, minced
- Fresh dill, chopped
- Olive oil
- Salt and pepper to taste

Instructions:

1. Preheat the oven to 400°F (200°C).
2. Place each salmon fillet on a piece of foil.
3. Arrange asparagus around the salmon.
4. Drizzle olive oil, sprinkle minced garlic, and season with salt and pepper.
5. Add lemon slices and fresh dill.
6. Seal the foil packets and bake for 20 minutes.

Nutritional Information:

- Calories: 380
- Protein: 35g
- Fat: 22g
- Carbohydrates: 10g
- Fiber: 4g / Sugar: 3g

27. Spinach and Artichoke Cauliflower Casserole (Low-Carb Comfort)

Ingredients:

- 1 head cauliflower, cut into florets
- Fresh spinach, chopped
- Artichoke hearts, drained and chopped
- Cream cheese
- Mozzarella cheese, shredded
- Garlic powder
- Salt and pepper to taste

Instructions:

1. Preheat the oven to 375°F (190°C).
2. Steam cauliflower until tender-crisp.
3. In a bowl, mix cauliflower with chopped spinach, artichoke hearts, cream cheese, and half of the mozzarella.
4. Season with garlic powder, salt, and pepper.
5. Transfer to a baking dish, top with the remaining mozzarella, and bake for 25-30 minutes.

Nutritional Information:

- Calories: 290
- Protein: 15g
- Fat: 20g
- Carbohydrates: 8g
- Fiber: 4g / Sugar: 3g

28. Turkey and Kale Soup (Hearty and Nutrient-Dense)

Ingredients:

- Ground turkey
- Kale, chopped
- Carrots, diced
- Celery, sliced
- Onion, diced
- Garlic, minced
- Low-sodium chicken broth
- Italian seasoning
- Salt and pepper to taste

Instructions:

1. In a pot, brown ground turkey with diced onion and minced garlic.
2. Add chopped kale, diced carrots, sliced celery, and low-sodium chicken broth.
3. Season with Italian seasoning, salt, and pepper.
4. Simmer for 20-25 minutes until vegetables are tender.

Nutritional Information:

- Calories: 250
- Protein: 20g
- Fat: 10g
- Carbohydrates: 15g
- Fiber: 5g / Sugar: 4g

29. Cucumber Avocado Salad (Cool and Refreshing)

Ingredients:

- Cucumbers, sliced
- Avocados, diced
- Cherry tomatoes, halved
- Red onion, thinly sliced
- Feta cheese, crumbled
- Olive oil
- Balsamic vinegar
- Fresh basil, chopped
- Salt and pepper to taste

Instructions:

1. In a bowl, combine sliced cucumbers, diced avocados, halved cherry tomatoes, thinly sliced red onion, and crumbled feta cheese.
2. Drizzle with olive oil and balsamic vinegar.
3. Sprinkle with fresh chopped basil, salt, and pepper.
4. Toss gently before serving.

Nutritional Information:

- Calories: 280
- Protein: 8g
- Fat: 22g
- Carbohydrates: 15g
- Fiber: 8g
- Sugar: 4g

30. Egg Drop Soup with Vegetables (Simple and Satisfying)

Ingredients:

- Chicken or vegetable broth (low-sodium)
- Eggs, beaten
- Mushrooms, sliced
- Green onions, chopped
- Soy sauce (low-sodium)
- Sesame oil
- Ginger, grated
- Sriracha (optional)

Instructions:

1. In a pot, bring low-sodium chicken or vegetable broth to a simmer.
2. Add sliced mushrooms and chopped green onions.
3. Drizzle beaten eggs into the simmering broth while stirring continuously.
4. Season with low-sodium soy sauce, sesame oil, and grated ginger.
5. Add a touch of Sriracha for extra heat if desired.

Nutritional Information:

- Calories: 180
- Protein: 12g
- Fat: 10g
- Carbohydrates: 8g
- Fiber: 2g
- Sugar: 3g

31. Greek Yogurt Parfait with Berries and Almonds (Protein-Packed Delight)

Ingredients:

- Greek yogurt
- Mixed berries (strawberries, blueberries, raspberries)
- Almonds, sliced
- Chia seeds
- Low-carb sweetener
- Vanilla extract

Instructions:

1. In a glass, layer Greek yogurt with mixed berries.
2. Sprinkle sliced almonds and chia seeds between the layers.
3. Drizzle with vanilla extract and a touch of low-carb sweetener.
4. Repeat the layers and top with additional berries.

Nutritional Information:

- Calories: 220
- Protein: 15g
- Fat: 12g
- Carbohydrates: 18g
- Fiber: 6g / Sugar: 8g

As you embark on this culinary journey, savor the richness of flavors, celebrate the diversity of ingredients, and relish the fact that Atkins allows you to tailor your meals to suit your unique tastes. With an array of recipes catering to every palate, Atkins becomes not just a diet but a delightful and sustainable way of eating that brings joy to your kitchen and vitality to your overall well-being.

CHAPTER EIGHT
THE 14-DAY REVITALIZATION PLAN: JUMPSTART YOUR JOURNEY

Embarking on a health and wellness journey can be both exciting and challenging, especially when you're eager to see quick and sustainable results. In this chapter, we'll delve into a comprehensive 14-day revitalization plan designed to jumpstart your transformation. Whether you're new to the Atkins lifestyle or looking to reinvigorate your commitment, this roadmap is tailored to deliver noticeable changes in just two weeks.

Your Two-Week Roadmap to Quick and Sustainable Results

Understanding the 14-Day Revitalization Plan

The first step in any transformative journey is clarity. In this section, we'll break down the core principles and objectives of the 14-day revitalization plan. By understanding the mechanics of this strategic roadmap, you'll be equipped with the knowledge needed to make informed choices and maximize the impact of this short-term commitment.

The 14-day plan is meticulously crafted to kickstart your metabolism, break through plateaus, and set the stage for long-term success. It combines the proven principles of the Atkins Diet with strategic meal planning and targeted activities to ignite your body's natural ability to burn fat. This isn't just a quick fix; it's a strategic approach to pave the way for sustained wellness.

Week 1: Priming Your Body for Change

Resetting and Rebalancing

The first week is dedicated to resetting and rebalancing your body. This involves a shift in dietary patterns, focusing on whole, nutrient-dense foods while eliminating potential culprits that might hinder your progress. Expect to see a reduction in carb intake during this phase, signaling your body to switch from using glucose as its primary fuel source to tapping into stored fat for energy.

Strategic Meal Planning: Nourishing Your Cells

During Week 1, we'll explore a diverse range of nutrient-rich recipes that not only align with the Atkins principles but also cater to your taste preferences. These meals are strategically crafted to provide essential vitamins, minerals, and antioxidants, giving your cells the nourishment they need to function optimally.

Incorporating Physical Activity: Moving with Purpose

To complement the dietary changes, Week 1 introduces purposeful physical activities tailored to your fitness level. Whether it's brisk walks, bodyweight exercises, or yoga sessions, these activities are designed to stimulate your metabolism, enhance circulation, and kickstart the fat-burning process.

Week 2: Accelerating Your Transformation

Intensifying the Atkins Advantage

As you transition into Week 2, the focus shifts to intensifying the Atkins advantage. This involves fine-tuning your macronutrient balance to optimize fat burning while maintaining a sense of satiety. The gradual reintroduction of certain foods allows for a more sustainable approach while keeping your body in a fat-burning state.

Fine-Tuning Your Macros: A Deeper Dive

Week 2 introduces a more nuanced approach to macronutrients, ensuring you strike the right balance between fats, proteins, and carbohydrates. We'll explore how adjusting these ratios can impact energy levels, cravings, and the overall effectiveness of the Atkins approach. This phase is about personalization, acknowledging that each individual's journey is unique.

Exploring Advanced Atkins Principles: Beyond the Basics

Building on the foundational principles of the Atkins Diet, Week 2 delves into advanced strategies that go beyond the basics. We'll explore concepts such as intermittent fasting, targeted supplementation, and mindful eating. These tools are designed to amplify your results and empower you with a deeper understanding of your body's responses to different stimuli.

Reflection and Adaptation: Beyond the 14 Days

Assessing Progress and Charting Your Course

As you approach the end of the 14-day revitalization plan, it's crucial to take a moment for reflection. This section guides you through assessing your progress, celebrating achievements, and acknowledging areas for further growth. Whether you've experienced significant weight loss, increased energy, or improved mental clarity, this reflective phase sets the stage for continued success.

Celebrating Milestones: Acknowledging Achievements

Take the time to celebrate both small and significant milestones achieved during the 14-day journey. Whether it's shedding a few pounds, breaking through a fitness barrier, or simply feeling more energized, these victories are the building blocks of your wellness transformation. Acknowledging your achievements boosts motivation and reinforces positive habits.

Adapting for Long-Term Success: Creating Your Blueprint

The 14-day revitalization plan is not a one-size-fits-all solution. In this final phase, we guide you through the process of adapting the lessons learned and strategies employed during this period into a sustainable long-term blueprint. This involves crafting an individualized approach that aligns with your lifestyle, preferences, and health goals.

In concluding the 14-day revitalization plan, it's essential to recognize that this journey is a springboard to lasting change. The principles, habits, and insights gained during this short but intense period will serve as a foundation for your ongoing wellness adventure. Whether you choose to continue with Atkins or integrate these lessons into your preferred lifestyle, the 14-day plan is a catalyst for transformative and sustainable change. Embrace the revitalized version of yourself and stride confidently into a future of vibrant well-being.

14-Day Metabolism-Boosting Atkins Meal Plan for Women Over 60

Nourishing Your Ageless Vitality

This meticulously crafted 14-day meal plan is specifically tailored for women over 60 following the Atkins Diet. Carefully designed to kickstart your metabolism, promote weight loss, and support overall well-being, each day offers a combination of nutrient-dense foods, delicious recipes, and the proven principles of Atkins to ensure a vibrant and ageless journey towards optimal health.

Day 1: Resetting with Flavorful Beginnings

Breakfast:

- Veggie omelette with mushrooms, spinach, and feta
- Sliced avocado on the side

Lunch:

- Chicken salad with mixed greens, cherry tomatoes, and a vinaigrette dressing

Dinner:

- Baked salmon with lemon and dill
- Cauliflower mash

Snack Options:

- Handful of nuts
- Greek yogurt with a sprinkle of chia seeds

Day 2: Embracing Wholesome Choices

Breakfast:

- Cottage cheese and berry bowl with a drizzle of honey

Lunch:

- Zucchini noodles with grilled chicken and pesto

Dinner:

- Turkey and vegetable stir-fry with broccoli and bell peppers
- Cauliflower rice

Snack Options:

- Sliced cucumber with tzatziki
- Hard-boiled eggs

Day 3: Low-Carb Delights for Longevity

Breakfast:

- Almond flour pancakes with fresh berries and sugar-free syrup

Lunch:

- Caprese salad with mozzarella, tomatoes, and basil
- Grilled shrimp on the side

Dinner:

- Beef and broccoli stir-fry
- Mashed sweet potatoes

Snack Options:

- Cheese and cherry tomato skewers
- Yogurt-covered almonds

Day 4: Protein-Packed Pleasures for Strength

Breakfast:

- Scrambled eggs with smoked salmon
- Avocado slices

Lunch:

- Chicken Caesar salad with extra parmesan and grilled chicken

Dinner:

- Baked cod fillets with garlic and herbs
- Steamed asparagus

Snack Options:

- Sliced bell peppers with hummus
- Protein smoothie with almond milk

Day 5: Balancing Macros for Resilience

Breakfast:

- Greek yogurt parfait with mixed berries and a sprinkle of granola

Lunch:

- Turkey and avocado wrap with whole-grain tortilla

Dinner:

- Eggplant lasagna with ground turkey
- Mixed green salad with olive oil dressing

Snack Options:

- Guacamole with celery sticks
- Mixed nuts and seeds trail mix

Day 6: Vibrant Vegetarian Delights

Breakfast:

- Spinach and feta omelette
- Tomato slices on the side

Lunch:

- Lentil and vegetable curry with quinoa

Dinner:

- Stuffed bell peppers with cauliflower rice
- Roasted Brussels sprouts

Snack Options:

- Celery sticks with almond butter
- Chia seed pudding with coconut milk

Day 7: Savoring Sunday Wellness

Breakfast:

- Whole grain toast with smashed avocado and poached eggs

Lunch:

- Shrimp and avocado salad with a tangy lime vinaigrette

Dinner:

- Grilled steak with garlic butter
- Mashed cauliflower

Snack Options:

- Fresh fruit skewers
- Cottage cheese with sliced peaches

Day 8: Fine-Tuning Macros for Aging Gracefully

Breakfast:

- Protein smoothie with spinach, banana, and almond milk

Lunch:

- Turkey and kale salad with a lemon-tahini dressing

Dinner:

- Baked chicken thighs with rosemary and lemon
- Sautéed green beans

Snack Options:

- Roasted chickpeas
- Mozzarella and cherry tomato bites

Day 9: Advanced Atkins Principles for Enhanced Wellness

Breakfast:

- Chia seed pudding with almond milk and a handful of raspberries

Lunch:

- Grilled salmon Caesar salad with extra parmesan

Dinner:

- Egg drop soup with vegetables and tofu
- Cauliflower fried rice

Snack Options:

- Apple slices with almond butter
- Hard-boiled eggs with a sprinkle of salt

Day 10: Variety in Vegetables for Nourishment

Breakfast:

- Whole grain toast with scrambled eggs and sautéed spinach

Lunch:

- Chickpea and vegetable stir-fry with tofu

Dinner:

- Baked tilapia with mango salsa
- Roasted Brussels sprouts

Snack Options:

- Cottage cheese with pineapple
- Mixed nuts and dried berries

Day 11: Tailoring the Journey to Your Taste

Breakfast:

- Almond flour blueberry muffins

Lunch:

- Turkey and avocado lettuce wraps with a light dressing

Dinner:

- Pork tenderloin with mustard glaze
- Grilled asparagus

Snack Options:

- Guacamole with carrot sticks

- Protein balls with cocoa and nuts

Day 12: Nutrient-Rich Indulgence for Sustained Energy

Breakfast:

- Greek yogurt smoothie with mixed berries and a scoop of protein powder

Lunch:

- Spinach and artichoke cauliflower casserole

Dinner:

- Grilled chicken thighs with pesto
- Zucchini noodles

Snack Options:

- Sliced cucumber with tzatziki
- Dark chocolate squares for a delightful treat

Day 13: Culinary Adventure Continues for Joyful Eating

Breakfast:

- Breakfast burrito with scrambled eggs, black beans, and salsa

Lunch:

- Caprese-stuffed avocados with balsamic glaze

Dinner:

- Beef and vegetable stir-fry with broccoli and snap peas
- Cauliflower rice

Snack Options:

- Yogurt-covered berries for a sweet touch
- Pumpkin seeds and dried apricots

Day 14: Celebrating Success and Renewed Vitality

Breakfast:

- Berry and protein-packed smoothie bowl with coconut flakes

Lunch:

- Tuna salad lettuce wraps with a squeeze of lemon

Dinner:

- Grilled shrimp skewers with garlic and herbs

- Mashed butternut squash

Snack Options:

- Cottage cheese with sliced strawberries

- Veggie chips with guacamole

As you conclude this 14-day metabolism-boosting Atkins meal plan, celebrate your renewed vitality and embrace the principles of the Atkins Diet for a sustained ageless lifestyle. May each nutrient-packed meal be a testament to your commitment to health and longevity. Continue savoring the flavors of wellness as you stride confidently into a future of vibrant well-being.

Overcoming Common Challenges in the Initial Phase

The initial phase of any health and wellness plan can be both exhilarating and challenging. As you commit to the 14-day revitalization plan, understanding the dynamics of this initial phase is crucial for setting realistic expectations and overcoming potential hurdles.

One common challenge faced during the initial phase is the body's adjustment to a new dietary routine. As you transition to the principles of the Atkins Diet, your metabolism undergoes a shift from utilizing primarily carbohydrates to tapping into stored fats for energy. This transition, often referred to as the "induction phase," may bring about what is commonly known as the "keto flu." Symptoms may include fatigue, headaches, and irritability as your body adapts to the metabolic shift.

To navigate this phase successfully, it's essential to stay hydrated, replenish electrolytes, and incorporate foods rich in potassium and magnesium. Additionally, recognizing that these symptoms are temporary and part of the body's adjustment process can help you stay motivated during this initial challenge.

Setting Realistic Expectations: Redefining Success

In the fervor of embarking on a 14-day revitalization plan, it's natural to have high expectations for rapid and significant changes. However, setting realistic expectations is key to maintaining motivation and achieving lasting success.

One challenge individuals often face is expecting drastic weight loss within the first few days. While initial weight loss may occur due to water weight reduction, sustainable fat loss takes time. It's crucial to shift the focus from the scale alone to overall well-being. Celebrate non-scale victories such as increased energy levels, improved mood, and better sleep quality.

Setting realistic goals is fundamental to long-term success. Instead of fixating on a specific weight target within the 14 days, consider goals like establishing a consistent exercise routine, incorporating diverse and nutrient-rich foods, and cultivating a positive mindset. By redefining success beyond the scale, you empower yourself to embrace the holistic nature of the revitalization journey.

Navigating Social and Emotional Challenges: The Power of Support

Embarking on a revitalization plan often involves navigating social and emotional challenges, as dietary changes can impact daily routines and social interactions. The support of friends and family plays a crucial role in overcoming these challenges.

One common concern is the pressure to conform to social norms, particularly during gatherings or events centered around food. Communicating your dietary choices with loved ones and explaining the purpose behind your 14-day plan fosters understanding and support. In many cases, friends and family may even join you on the journey, creating a shared commitment to health.

Emotional challenges, such as stress eating or using food as a coping mechanism, may also surface during the initial phase. Developing alternative strategies to manage stress, such as practicing mindfulness, engaging in physical activity, or seeking emotional support, is vital. The revitalization plan is not just about transforming your body but also nurturing a positive relationship with food and emotions.

Fine-Tuning Your Meal Plan: Adapting to Preferences and Tastes

Crafting a meal plan that aligns with your taste preferences is a pivotal aspect of the 14-day revitalization journey. Fine-tuning your meals to suit your palate not only enhances satisfaction but also ensures long-term adherence to the plan.

One challenge faced in the initial phase is finding a balance between following the prescribed guidelines and personalizing your meals. The key is to view the revitalization plan as a flexible framework rather than a rigid set of rules. While adhering to the core principles of the Atkins Diet, feel empowered to make choices that cater to your taste preferences.

Experimenting with diverse recipes, incorporating herbs and spices for added flavor, and exploring different cooking methods can transform your meals into a delightful culinary experience. By embracing variety and flexibility, you not only make the revitalization plan more enjoyable but also lay the foundation for sustained wellness beyond the 14 days.

Overcoming Plateaus: Strategies for Continuous Progress

The initial enthusiasm of a revitalization plan can sometimes be met with plateaus, where progress appears to stall. Overcoming plateaus requires a strategic approach that goes beyond the dietary aspect and encompasses various elements of your well-being.

One common challenge is the initial rapid weight loss, followed by a period where the scale seems unyielding. It's essential to recognize that weight loss is not always linear, and plateaus are a natural part of the journey. Instead of becoming disheartened, focus on non-scale victories, such as improved fitness levels, enhanced mental clarity, and clothing fitting more comfortably.

To overcome plateaus, consider introducing variety into your exercise routine, reassessing portion sizes, and incorporating intermittent fasting. Additionally, ensuring adequate sleep and managing stress levels can positively impact your body's response to the revitalization plan. By adopting a holistic approach, you break through plateaus and foster continuous progress.

Staying Motivated: Cultivating a Positive Mindset

Maintaining motivation throughout the 14-day revitalization plan is integral to its success. Cultivating a positive mindset involves acknowledging achievements, learning from challenges, and embracing the transformative nature of the journey.

A common challenge individuals face is the temptation to revert to old habits when faced with setbacks. Instead of viewing challenges as failures, perceive them as opportunities for growth and refinement. Celebrate small victories, whether it's resisting an unhealthy snack or completing a challenging workout.

Staying motivated also involves visualizing your goals and envisioning the positive outcomes of the revitalization plan. Create a vision board, journal your progress, and surround yourself with affirmations that reinforce your commitment to health. By fostering a positive mindset, you not only navigate challenges more effectively but also set the stage for sustained motivation beyond the 14 days.

As you navigate the initial phase of the 14-day revitalization plan, remember that challenges are stepping stones to success. Understanding, adapting, and staying motivated empower you to overcome hurdles and emerge victorious in your journey towards revitalized well-being. The 14 days are not just a countdown but a transformative experience that lays the foundation for a healthier and more vibrant you.

Celebrating Successes and Navigating Setbacks With Resilience

Embarking on a revitalization journey involves more than just physical transformation—it's a holistic process that demands reflection, resilience, and a celebration of both successes and setbacks. In this chapter, we delve into the importance of acknowledging achievements, navigating setbacks with resilience, and maintaining the momentum towards your health and wellness goals.

Celebrating Successes: Acknowledging Milestones

As you progress through the 14-day revitalization plan, taking the time to celebrate your successes is not just a form of self-indulgence; it's a crucial aspect of sustaining motivation and building confidence in your journey.

One key success to celebrate is adherence to the dietary guidelines. Whether you've successfully embraced low-carb meals, increased your water intake, or navigated social challenges, these milestones deserve recognition. Celebrate your commitment to change and the positive impact it's having on your overall well-being.

Physical achievements, such as improved energy levels, better sleep, or increased stamina, are also worth acknowledging. Remember that success extends beyond the number on the scale. Celebrate every positive change, big or small, as they collectively contribute to the transformative process.

Navigating Setbacks: Learning from Challenges

In any transformative journey, setbacks are inevitable. Navigating these setbacks with resilience and a growth mindset is key to maintaining forward momentum. Instead of viewing setbacks as failures, consider them as opportunities for learning and refinement.

One common setback is facing unexpected challenges that disrupt your routine, such as a hectic work schedule or family obligations. Rather than abandoning your revitalization plan, use these challenges as opportunities to adapt. Quick, convenient meal options and incorporating short, intense workouts can help you stay on track during busy times.

Another setback individuals often encounter is the temptation to revert to old habits, especially in moments of stress or emotional upheaval. Developing alternative coping mechanisms, such as mindfulness, meditation, or engaging in a hobby, empowers you to navigate emotional challenges without compromising your progress.

Resilience in the Face of Adversity: Building Inner Strength

Building resilience is not just about bouncing back from setbacks; it's about developing inner strength to withstand the challenges that come your way. Resilience is the bedrock of sustained well-being, and its cultivation is integral to the success of the 14-day revitalization plan.

One aspect of resilience is the ability to adapt to change. Embracing a revitalization plan involves a shift in lifestyle, and adaptation is a continuous process. Rather than resisting change, cultivate a mindset of flexibility and openness. Remember, each challenge is an opportunity for growth.

Maintaining resilience also involves cultivating a strong support system. Share your journey with friends, family, or a community following a similar path. The collective strength of a supportive network can be a powerful motivator during challenging times. Don't hesitate to seek guidance or encouragement when needed.

Mindfulness and Reflection: Nurturing Self-Awareness

Amidst the whirlwind of a revitalization plan, incorporating mindfulness and reflection practices can provide a valuable anchor. Mindfulness allows you to stay present in the moment, fostering a deeper connection with your choices and actions.

One setback many individuals face is mindless eating—an automatic response to external stimuli or emotions. Mindfulness practices, such as mindful eating, bring awareness to the act of consuming food. Chew slowly, savor each bite, and listen to your body's signals of hunger and satiety. This mindful approach helps you make conscious choices aligned with your revitalization goals.

Reflection is another potent tool for self-awareness. Regularly journaling your experiences, challenges, and triumphs provides clarity on your journey. Consider creating a daily log to track your meals, emotions, and physical activities. This reflective process enhances self-awareness and strengthens your commitment to the revitalization plan.

Reassessing Goals: Adapting to Evolving Priorities

As you progress through the 14-day revitalization plan, reassessing your goals becomes paramount. Your initial objectives may have evolved, and adapting them to align with your current priorities ensures continued motivation and relevance.

One common setback is feeling demotivated when the initial excitement wanes. Reassessing your goals allows you to realign them with your evolving priorities, preventing stagnation. Perhaps your focus shifts from weight loss to overall well-being, or from external validation to cultivating intrinsic motivation.

Celebrate the goals you've achieved, no matter how small, and use them as stepping stones for setting new ones. Whether it's incorporating a new type of exercise, exploring diverse low-carb recipes, or enhancing your mindfulness practices, adapt your goals to keep the revitalization journey dynamic and engaging.

Building a Sustainable Lifestyle: Beyond the 14 Days

The ultimate success of the 14-day revitalization plan lies in its ability to lay the foundation for a sustainable lifestyle. Instead of viewing the plan as a short-term fix, consider it a catalyst for long-lasting changes that extend far beyond the initial two weeks.

One setback individuals often encounter is the temptation to revert to old habits once the 14 days conclude. To overcome this, transition into a maintenance phase that integrates the principles of the revitalization plan into your daily life. Gradually reintroduce certain foods while monitoring their impact on your well-being.

Building a sustainable lifestyle also involves ongoing education and self-discovery. Stay informed about nutrition, fitness, and holistic well-being. Experiment with different foods, exercises, and mindfulness practices to discover what works best for you. The revitalization plan is a launchpad for continuous growth and refinement.

A Journey of Resilience and Celebration

As you navigate the complexities of the 14-day revitalization plan, remember that the journey is not just about the destination; it's about the resilience you build and the successes you celebrate along the way. Embrace setbacks as opportunities for growth, cultivate resilience, and let the journey unfold as a celebration of your commitment to lasting well-being. The 14 days are merely the beginning of a transformative lifestyle that honors your health and vitality.

CHAPTER NINE
NAVIGATING HEALTH CHALLENGES:
ATKINS SOLUTIONS

Navigating health challenges requires a holistic approach that encompasses dietary choices, lifestyle modifications, and a nuanced understanding of the relationship between nutrition and chronic conditions. In this chapter, we delve into how Atkins offers a synergistic approach to managing chronic conditions, paving the way for enhanced well-being and vitality.

Atkins and Chronic Conditions: A Synergistic Approach

Managing chronic conditions necessitates a comprehensive strategy that addresses not only symptoms but also the underlying factors contributing to the condition. The Atkins Diet, known for its low-carbohydrate approach, has shown promise in synergizing with conventional medical interventions to manage various chronic conditions.

One of the primary benefits of the Atkins Diet is its impact on insulin sensitivity. For individuals with conditions like type 2 diabetes, insulin resistance is a key concern. The low-carb nature of the Atkins Diet helps regulate blood sugar levels, reducing the strain on insulin-producing cells. Research suggests that following a low-carbohydrate diet can lead to improved glycemic control, making it a valuable tool in the management of diabetes.

Additionally, the Atkins Diet has demonstrated effectiveness in supporting weight management, a crucial aspect of addressing conditions such as hypertension and metabolic syndrome. Excess weight can exacerbate these conditions, and the controlled carbohydrate intake in the Atkins approach has been associated with weight loss and improved cardiovascular health.

Tailoring Atkins to Specific Conditions: Personalized Wellness Plans

The beauty of the Atkins approach lies in its adaptability to different health needs. Tailoring the Atkins Diet to specific chronic conditions involves creating personalized wellness plans that consider individual health goals, dietary preferences, and medical recommendations.

For individuals with cardiovascular conditions, a modified Atkins Diet that prioritizes heart-healthy fats, lean proteins, and fiber-rich vegetables can be beneficial. This approach not only supports cardiovascular health but also aligns with dietary recommendations for conditions like hyperlipidemia.

In the case of autoimmune conditions, where inflammation plays a significant role, the anti-inflammatory potential of the Atkins Diet can be harnessed. Emphasizing foods with anti-inflammatory properties, such as fatty fish, olive oil, and leafy greens, may contribute to managing symptoms and promoting overall well-being.

Supporting Cognitive Health: Atkins and Neurological Conditions

Cognitive health is a vital aspect of overall wellness, and certain chronic conditions, such as Alzheimer's disease, present unique challenges. The role of nutrition in supporting cognitive function is gaining attention, and the Atkins Diet's potential impact on neurological conditions is an area of ongoing research.

The brain's reliance on glucose for energy raises questions about the compatibility of low-carbohydrate diets with cognitive health. However, emerging studies suggest that ketones, produced during the breakdown of fats in a low-carb state, may serve as an alternative energy source for the brain. This metabolic flexibility is being explored as a potential avenue for supporting cognitive function.

While more research is needed in this area, the Atkins approach, with its focus on healthy fats, lean proteins, and non-starchy vegetables, aligns with general dietary recommendations for cognitive health. Moreover, the potential benefits of ketones in neurological conditions underscore the importance of personalized approaches and ongoing medical supervision.

Atkins and Inflammation: A Balancing Act for Immune Health

Inflammation is a common denominator in many chronic conditions, from arthritis to inflammatory bowel diseases. The Atkins Diet's impact on inflammation is a subject of interest, as certain dietary components can either fuel or mitigate inflammatory processes.

The low-carbohydrate, high-fat nature of the Atkins approach has shown promise in reducing markers of inflammation. By minimizing the intake of refined carbohydrates and processed foods, individuals may experience a decrease in inflammatory responses. This is particularly relevant for conditions where chronic inflammation plays a role in disease progression.

Moreover, the inclusion of anti-inflammatory foods within the Atkins framework, such as fatty fish, nuts, and colorful vegetables, provides a balanced approach to immune health. The emphasis on nutrient-dense, whole foods complements the goal of managing inflammation and fostering overall well-being.

Addressing Gut Health: Atkins and Gastrointestinal Conditions

Gut health is intricately linked to overall wellness, and conditions like irritable bowel syndrome (IBS) and inflammatory bowel diseases require a nuanced dietary approach. The Atkins Diet's focus on whole foods and the potential impact on gut health make it a candidate for individuals navigating gastrointestinal conditions.

The controlled carbohydrate intake in the Atkins approach may offer relief to individuals with IBS, where certain carbohydrates can trigger symptoms. By emphasizing non-starchy vegetables, lean proteins, and healthy fats, individuals can tailor their Atkins plans to support gut-friendly eating.

Moreover, the inclusion of probiotic-rich foods within the Atkins framework, such as yogurt and fermented vegetables, aligns with recommendations for promoting a healthy gut microbiome. Emerging research suggests that the composition of gut bacteria plays a role in gastrointestinal conditions, and the Atkins approach provides a flexible platform for individuals to explore dietary strategies that support their unique needs.

Safety and Consultation: Navigating Atkins with Medical Guidance

While the Atkins Diet shows promise in supporting various aspects of health, it's crucial to approach dietary changes, especially for chronic conditions, with medical guidance. Safety and individualization are paramount to ensure that the Atkins approach aligns with specific medical needs and goals.

Before embarking on an Atkins journey, individuals with chronic conditions should consult with healthcare professionals, including physicians, registered dietitians, or specialists relevant to their condition. Medical supervision ensures a thorough understanding of the individual's health status, medications, and potential interactions with dietary changes.

Additionally, healthcare professionals can provide valuable insights into tailoring the Atkins Diet to specific conditions, adjusting macronutrient ratios, and monitoring potential changes in health parameters. Regular check-ins and collaboration between individuals and their healthcare team contribute to a holistic and safe approach to managing chronic conditions with the Atkins Diet.

Empowering Wellness Through Personalized Solutions

Navigating health challenges with the Atkins Diet involves recognizing the synergistic potential between dietary choices and chronic conditions. By embracing personalized wellness plans, tailoring the Atkins approach to specific health needs, and seeking medical guidance, individuals can empower their journey towards enhanced well-being. The Atkins Diet becomes not just a dietary plan but a versatile tool in the broader landscape of holistic health management.

Managing Health Concerns Through Strategic Dietary Choices

The Power of Strategic Dietary Choices

In the intricate tapestry of health challenges, strategic dietary choices stand as a beacon of empowerment. This chapter explores the profound impact of the Atkins Diet on managing health concerns, providing a roadmap for individuals to navigate the complexities of their well-being through intentional and strategic nutrition.

Understanding The Role of Nutrition: A Foundation For Health

To comprehend the profound influence of the Atkins Diet on health concerns, it's essential to first grasp the pivotal role that nutrition plays in overall well-being. The food we consume serves as the building blocks for our bodies, influencing everything from energy levels to immune function.

Nutrition is not merely a means of satisfying hunger; it is a dynamic interplay of nutrients that regulate physiological processes. The strategic manipulation of these nutrients through the Atkins Diet becomes a powerful tool for managing health concerns. By understanding the intricate dance between carbohydrates, fats, and proteins, individuals can tailor their dietary choices to address specific health needs.

Strategic Carbohydrate Management: Balancing Energy and Wellness

At the heart of the Atkins approach lies the strategic management of carbohydrates—a key element in the quest for overall health and wellness. Carbohydrates, while a primary source of energy, can pose challenges when consumed excessively or in the form of refined and processed foods.

The Atkins Diet strategically addresses carbohydrate intake by categorizing them into different phases. In the initial phase, known as induction, carbohydrate intake is significantly reduced to promote a state of ketosis. This metabolic shift encourages the body to burn stored fat for fuel, leading to weight loss and potential improvements in health markers.

As individuals progress through the phases, they reintroduce carbohydrates in a controlled manner, allowing for a customized approach that aligns with personal health goals. Strategic carbohydrate management not only supports weight management but also addresses concerns related to insulin resistance, metabolic syndrome, and type 2 diabetes.

Fats as Allies: Dispelling Myths and Embracing Healthy Fats

In the realm of health concerns, fats have often been misunderstood and wrongly vilified. The Atkins Diet challenges these misconceptions by emphasizing the importance of healthy fats as allies in the pursuit of well-being.

Contrary to the outdated notion that all fats are detrimental, the Atkins approach distinguishes between unhealthy trans fats and saturated fats and the beneficial unsaturated fats. Healthy fats play a crucial role in supporting various bodily functions, from hormone production to brain health.

By incorporating sources of healthy fats such as avocados, nuts, olive oil, and fatty fish, individuals can strategically enhance their nutritional profile. This strategic integration of fats not only supports overall health but also addresses concerns related to cardiovascular health, inflammation, and neurological well-being.

Protein Power: Nourishing the Body and Fostering Vitality

Protein, often hailed as the building block of life, takes center stage in the Atkins approach to managing health concerns. Beyond its role in muscle building, protein plays a multifaceted role in supporting immune function, satiety, and metabolic processes.

Strategic protein intake is a hallmark of the Atkins Diet, contributing to the preservation of lean muscle mass while promoting fat loss. This becomes particularly relevant in addressing concerns related to metabolic health, where maintaining a healthy body composition is pivotal.

Moreover, protein's satiating effect becomes a strategic tool in managing weight and supporting dietary adherence. By strategically incorporating protein-rich foods such as lean meats, poultry, eggs, and plant-based sources, individuals can navigate health concerns with a focus on sustained vitality.

Micronutrient Mastery: Unlocking the Power of Nutrient-Dense Foods

The strategic approach of the Atkins Diet extends beyond macronutrients to encompass the realm of micronutrients—essential vitamins and minerals that play a fundamental role in health. Micronutrient mastery involves consciously selecting nutrient-dense foods to address deficiencies and optimize overall well-being.

In managing health concerns, micronutrients act as catalysts for various physiological processes. For instance, adequate levels of vitamin D are crucial for bone health, while antioxidants like vitamin C and E play a role in combating oxidative stress and inflammation.

The Atkins Diet encourages the consumption of nutrient-dense vegetables, fruits, and other whole foods rich in vitamins and minerals. This strategic focus on micronutrient mastery ensures that individuals not only meet their macronutrient goals but also fortify their bodies with the essential elements necessary for robust health.

Hydration Harmony: The Overlooked Pillar of Well-Being

In the labyrinth of health concerns, hydration often emerges as an overlooked yet indispensable factor. The Atkins Diet strategically addresses the importance of hydration, recognizing its role in metabolic processes, toxin elimination, and overall vitality.

Adequate water intake becomes a strategic tool in managing health concerns, from supporting digestion to optimizing cognitive function. The Atkins approach encourages individuals to prioritize water consumption, especially during the initial phases where metabolic shifts may increase fluid needs.

Strategic hydration goes beyond quenching thirst; it becomes a cornerstone of well-being. By fostering hydration harmony through water-rich foods, herbal teas, and mindful fluid intake, individuals can navigate health concerns with a holistic approach that encompasses both macro and micronutrients.

Customizing Atkins for Personal Health Goals: A Strategic Roadmap

The power of the Atkins Diet lies in its inherent flexibility, allowing individuals to customize their approach based on personal health goals. This strategic customization involves a thoughtful integration of the Atkins principles into one's lifestyle, aligning dietary choices with specific health concerns.

For weight management, individuals may strategically focus on the phases that support fat loss while preserving lean muscle mass. Those with metabolic concerns can customize their Atkins approach to emphasize carbohydrate management and insulin sensitivity.

Furthermore, individuals navigating specific health concerns, such as autoimmune conditions or gastrointestinal issues, can tailor their dietary choices within the Atkins framework. This strategic customization ensures that the Atkins Diet becomes not just a generic plan but a personalized roadmap for addressing individual health needs.

Strategic Planning for Long-Term Success: Beyond Quick Fixes

In the realm of health concerns, the Atkins Diet distinguishes itself by fostering a strategic planning mindset focused on long-term success. Unlike quick-fix approaches that often lead to temporary results, the Atkins strategy involves sustained dietary choices that support ongoing well-being.

Strategic planning encompasses not only the immediate goals but also the evolving health landscape. Individuals are encouraged to view the Atkins Diet as a dynamic tool that can be adjusted to meet changing health needs. This involves periodic reassessments, consultations with healthcare professionals, and a commitment to lifelong learning about one's health.

By adopting a strategic planning perspective, individuals can navigate health concerns with resilience and adaptability. The Atkins approach becomes a companion in the journey towards enduring well-being, addressing not just the symptoms but the root causes of health concerns.

Empowering Health Through Strategic Nutrition

In the intricate dance of health challenges, strategic dietary choices emerge as a potent force for empowerment. The Atkins Diet, with its emphasis on strategic carbohydrate management, healthy fats, protein power, micronutrient mastery, hydration harmony, and customizable approaches, becomes a roadmap for individuals to navigate the complexities of their well-being. The chapter concludes with a call to embrace strategic nutrition as a cornerstone of a vibrant and resilient life.

Real-Life Stories: Women Over 60 Triumphing with Atkins

In the realm of real-life stories, the narratives of women over 60 triumphing with the Atkins Diet stand as powerful testimonies to the transformative potential of strategic dietary choices. These women, from diverse backgrounds and walks of life, share their journeys of resilience, empowerment, and vibrant living through the Atkins approach.

1. A Journey to Reclaim Vitality: Margaret's Story

Meet Margaret, a spirited woman in her early 60s who embarked on an Atkins journey to reclaim her vitality. Struggling with weight gain and feeling sluggish, Margaret sought a solution that aligned with her age and health considerations. Through strategic carbohydrate management and embracing healthy fats, Margaret not only shed excess pounds but also discovered a newfound energy that revitalized her daily life. Her story exemplifies how age is no barrier to transformation, and with the right dietary choices, vibrant living can be a reality.

2. Thriving After Menopause: Susan's Atkins Triumph

Susan, in her late 60s, faced the challenges of navigating menopause and its associated symptoms. Seeking a holistic approach, she turned to the Atkins Diet. By incorporating Atkins-friendly foods that supported hormonal stability, Susan experienced relief from hot flashes and improved overall well-being. Her journey highlights the role of strategic nutrition in managing life transitions, proving that women over 60 can thrive and triumph in the face of physiological changes.

3. Bone Health Resilience: Patricia's Atkins Success

Patricia, a vibrant woman in her 70s, prioritized bone health as a key aspect of her well-being. Recognizing the role of nutrition in bone health after 60, she tailored the Atkins principles to include a focus on nutrient-dense foods that support bone density. Through her commitment to the Atkins approach, Patricia not only strengthened her foundation but also inspired others to prioritize skeletal health in their wellness journeys. Her story illuminates the significance of personalized dietary choices in fortifying the body for long-term vitality.

4. Muscular Vitality Beyond 60: Carol's Atkins Adventure

Carol, in her late 60s, defied stereotypes by embracing resistance training and the Atkins Diet as a dynamic duo for muscular vitality. Through protein-packed perfection and a commitment to staying strong and active, Carol not only preserved her muscle mass but also discovered a newfound strength that transcended age expectations. Her real-life triumph exemplifies that building and

preserving muscle mass is not only possible but can become a fulfilling part of a woman's journey well into her 60s and beyond.

5. Diabetes Defense and Atkins: Linda's Inspiring Journey

Linda, navigating the complexities of diabetes in her mid-60s, found hope and empowerment through the Atkins approach. Understanding the connection between carbs and blood sugar, she crafted low-carb meals for stable blood sugar, taking control of her health. Linda's story sheds light on the empowering role of strategic dietary choices in diabetes prevention and management, proving that women over 60 can wield the Atkins principles as a powerful defense against the challenges of this condition.

These real-life stories of women over 60 triumphing with Atkins serve as beacons of inspiration for those embarking on their own wellness journeys. Through strategic dietary choices, these women have not only transformed their lives but also shattered preconceived notions about aging. As we delve into their triumphs, we are reminded that the Atkins Diet is more than a nutritional strategy—it is a catalyst for vibrant living, resilience, and embracing the next chapter with grace and vitality.

CHAPTER TEN
AGELESS VITALITY: ATKINS FOR A LIFETIME

In the pursuit of ageless vitality, the Atkins Diet emerges as a guiding light, offering a sustainable and transformative approach to nutrition. This chapter delves into the core principles that make Atkins a lifestyle for a lifetime, emphasizing the significance of sustaining progress and achieving long-term success.

Understanding Ageless Vitality: A Holistic Perspective

Ageless vitality is not a fleeting concept but a holistic state of being that encompasses physical well-being, mental clarity, and emotional resilience. The Atkins Diet, rooted in strategic nutrition, provides a holistic perspective on ageless vitality. By addressing the interplay of macronutrients, micronutrients, and lifestyle factors, individuals can embark on a journey that transcends the limitations often associated with aging. This section explores the foundational principles that form the bedrock of ageless vitality through the Atkins approach.

Sustaining Your Progress: Long-Term Atkins Success

Sustaining progress is the linchpin of ageless vitality, and the Atkins Diet excels in providing a roadmap for long-term success. This segment delves into the key strategies and mindset shifts necessary to navigate the various phases of the Atkins journey, ensuring that individuals not only achieve their initial goals but continue to thrive in the years to come.

Transitioning Through Phases: A Lifelong Approach

The Atkins Diet is not a one-size-fits-all solution; it's a customizable framework that evolves with individuals as they progress through different phases. Whether starting with the induction phase for rapid results or transitioning to a maintenance phase for sustainable living, the Atkins approach is designed to accommodate changing needs and goals. This section outlines the importance of understanding and embracing the transitional nature of the Atkins Diet for ageless vitality.

Embracing Flexibility: A Dynamic Lifestyle

Ageless vitality thrives on adaptability, and the Atkins lifestyle is inherently flexible. From tailoring the diet to individual preferences to incorporating diverse nutrient sources, flexibility is a cornerstone of long-term success. By emphasizing the dynamic nature of the Atkins approach, individuals can weave the principles into their daily lives, adapting to new challenges and opportunities without compromising their commitment to ageless vitality.

Building Lasting Habits: The Foundation of a Lifetime

Habits, once ingrained, become the building blocks of a lifetime. This section explores the psychology of habit formation and how the Atkins Diet encourages the development of sustainable, health-promoting habits. From mindful eating practices to incorporating regular physical activity, individuals learn to weave these habits into the fabric of their lives, contributing to ageless vitality that endures through the years.

Monitoring and Adjusting: A Proactive Approach

Ageless vitality requires a proactive stance toward health, and the Atkins Diet empowers individuals to monitor and adjust their approach as needed. Regular check-ins, self-assessment, and, when necessary, consultations with healthcare professionals ensure that the dietary choices align with evolving health needs. This segment underscores the importance of taking a proactive and informed approach to long-term success with the Atkins lifestyle.

Celebrating Milestones: Markers of Ageless Vitality

In the journey towards ageless vitality, celebrating milestones becomes a vital component. Whether it's achieving weight loss goals, overcoming health challenges, or simply experiencing a surge in energy and well-being, each milestone is a marker of success. This section explores the significance of acknowledging and celebrating these achievements, fostering a positive mindset that fuels continued commitment to the Atkins lifestyle.

Staying Connected: The Role of Community

The Atkins community becomes a valuable support system in the quest for ageless vitality. By staying connected with like-minded individuals, sharing experiences, and drawing inspiration from the collective journey, individuals strengthen their resolve and commitment. This section highlights the role of community support in sustaining progress, fostering a sense of belonging, and enriching the ageless vitality journey.

Culinary Adventures: Ageless Vitality on Your Plate

The kitchen becomes a canvas for ageless vitality, and this section explores the culinary adventures that the Atkins Diet offers. From exploring diverse low-carb recipes to experimenting with nutrient-dense ingredients, individuals discover the joy of crafting meals that not only nourish the body but also delight the palate. The intersection of ageless vitality and culinary creativity is celebrated as an integral aspect of the Atkins lifestyle.

This chapter reinforces the idea that ageless vitality is not a destination but a lifelong commitment. By internalizing the principles of sustained progress, embracing flexibility, building lasting habits, proactively monitoring health, celebrating milestones, and staying connected, individuals can weave the Atkins approach into the fabric of their lives. The chapter closes with an invitation to embark on a journey towards ageless vitality that transcends the boundaries of time, enabling individuals to thrive in every chapter of their lives.

Staying Energetic, Healthy, and Happy Beyond 60

Ageless vitality is more than a concept; it's a lifestyle approach that encapsulates staying energetic, healthy, and happy beyond the age of 60. The Atkins Diet, with its strategic nutrition principles, emerges as a key ally in this journey. This chapter delves into the strategies and insights that can empower individuals to cultivate ageless vitality and embrace the richness of life well into their senior years.

Understanding Ageless Vitality: A Holistic Approach

Ageless vitality isn't just about the absence of illness but a comprehensive state of well-being that encompasses physical vibrancy, mental clarity, and emotional equilibrium. The Atkins Diet serves as a catalyst for this holistic approach, recognizing the interplay between nutrition, lifestyle, and overall vitality. This section sets the stage for exploring the key elements that contribute to staying energetic, healthy, and happy beyond the age of 60.

Staying Energetic: The Role of Nutrition and Lifestyle

Strategic Carbohydrate Management for Sustained Energy

One of the pillars of ageless vitality is sustained energy, and strategic carbohydrate management lies at the heart of achieving this goal. The Atkins Diet, known for its controlled carbohydrate approach, helps regulate blood sugar levels, preventing energy crashes often associated with high-carb diets. By emphasizing low-glycemic foods and incorporating complex carbohydrates, individuals can maintain a steady supply of energy throughout the day, promoting vitality and resilience.

Protein Power and Muscle Preservation

Age-related muscle loss can contribute to a decline in energy levels. The Atkins Diet, with its emphasis on protein power, becomes a strategic tool for preserving lean muscle mass. Adequate protein intake supports muscle maintenance and repair, ensuring that individuals can sustain their energy levels and physical strength as they age. This section explores the synergy between protein-rich nutrition and sustained energy, fostering a vibrant and energetic lifestyle.

Hydration Harmony for Physical Vitality

Dehydration can sap energy and contribute to feelings of fatigue. In the quest for ageless vitality, hydration harmony plays a pivotal role. The Atkins approach encourages individuals to prioritize water intake, ensuring proper hydration to support metabolic processes and overall physical vitality. By incorporating water-rich foods and adopting mindful hydration practices, individuals can safeguard their energy levels and promote a vibrant, active lifestyle.

Promoting Health Beyond 60: A Nutritional Blueprint

Navigating Age-Related Health Challenges

As individuals age, they may encounter specific health challenges that require a nuanced nutritional approach. The Atkins Diet provides a blueprint for promoting health beyond 60 by addressing common concerns such as metabolic changes, bone health, and cardiovascular wellness. Through tailored nutrition plans that focus on nutrient-dense foods and targeted supplementation when needed, individuals can navigate age-related health challenges and proactively support their overall well-being.

Anti-Inflammatory Nutrition for Joint Health

Inflammation, often associated with aging, can impact joint health and contribute to discomfort. The Atkins approach, with its emphasis on anti-inflammatory nutrition, becomes a valuable tool in promoting joint health beyond 60. By incorporating foods rich in omega-3 fatty acids, antioxidants, and anti-inflammatory compounds, individuals can mitigate inflammation, support joint function, and enhance their overall physical well-being.

Balancing Hormones Through Smart Nutrition

Hormonal imbalances are common as individuals age, impacting various aspects of health. The Atkins Diet acknowledges the role of hormones in overall vitality and provides a framework for balancing hormones through smart nutrition. By incorporating hormone-supportive foods and optimizing macronutrient ratios, individuals can foster hormonal harmony, promoting not only physical health but also emotional well-being.

Cultivating Happiness in the Golden Years

The Gut-Brain Connection: Nutrition for Cognitive Health

Happiness in the golden years goes beyond physical well-being; cognitive health plays a crucial role. The Atkins Diet, with its focus on the gut-brain connection, recognizes the impact of nutrition on cognitive function. By prioritizing foods that support a healthy gut microbiome, individuals can positively influence their mood, cognitive abilities, and overall mental well-being. This section explores the intersection of nutrition and cognitive health, contributing to a holistic approach to happiness in the golden years.

Mindful Eating and Emotional Resilience

Ageless vitality encompasses emotional resilience, and mindful eating becomes a key practice in cultivating happiness. The Atkins approach encourages individuals to be mindful of their food choices, savoring each bite and fostering a positive relationship with food. By avoiding emotional eating patterns and embracing mindful eating practices, individuals can enhance their emotional well-being, promoting happiness and contentment as they age.

Embracing the Full Spectrum of Life

In conclusion, ageless vitality with Atkins goes beyond a dietary plan—it's a lifestyle that empowers individuals to stay energetic, healthy, and happy beyond 60. By understanding the holistic nature of ageless vitality, incorporating strategic nutrition and lifestyle choices, and cultivating happiness in the golden years, individuals can embrace the full spectrum of life with vigor and enthusiasm. The chapter closes with an invitation to embark on this transformative journey towards ageless vitality, celebrating the richness that each stage of life brings.

Your Personal Atkins Toolkit for A Lifelong Health Adventure

Ageless vitality requires more than a one-size-fits-all solution; it demands a personalized approach that adapts to the unique needs and goals of each individual. This chapter explores how you can build your personal Atkins toolkit—a comprehensive set of strategies, habits, and mindset shifts that will guide you through a lifelong health adventure, ensuring sustained well-being and vitality.

Understanding Your Personal Health Adventure: A Holistic View

Embarking on a lifelong health adventure requires a holistic perspective that considers every facet of your well-being. The Atkins Diet, with its multifaceted approach, becomes the foundation for crafting your personal toolkit. This section introduces the concept of a lifelong health adventure, emphasizing the interconnectedness of nutrition, lifestyle, and mindset in achieving ageless vitality.

Building a Foundation: Key Principles of Your Atkins Toolkit

Strategic Carbohydrate Management: The Core Principle

At the heart of your personal Atkins toolkit lies the core principle of strategic carbohydrate management. Understanding how different carbohydrates impact your body and tailoring your intake to match your health goals becomes a foundational strategy. Whether you're in the initial phases focusing on weight loss or maintaining your progress in later stages, this principle remains pivotal in sustaining energy, managing weight, and supporting overall vitality.

Protein Power and Lean Muscle Maintenance

Protein is your ally in preserving lean muscle mass, supporting metabolic functions, and ensuring long-term health. Your personal toolkit emphasizes the importance of incorporating protein-rich foods, understanding your unique protein needs, and leveraging protein's satiating effect to enhance overall satisfaction with your dietary choices.

Healthy Fats for Cognitive Health and Vitality

In your health adventure, healthy fats play a crucial role in promoting cognitive health, supporting cardiovascular well-being, and contributing to overall vitality. Your toolkit guides you in identifying sources of healthy fats, striking a balance between different types of fats, and appreciating the diverse benefits they bring to your ageless vitality journey.

Micronutrient Mastery: A Nutrient-Rich Approach

A key component of your toolkit is mastering the art of micronutrients—essential vitamins and minerals that fuel various physiological processes. Your personalized approach involves selecting nutrient-dense foods, understanding the role of specific micronutrients in your health, and ensuring that your diet is rich in the elements that contribute to sustained well-being.

Customizing Your Toolkit: Tailoring Atkins to Your Unique Needs

Phased Approach for Lifelong Success

Your personal toolkit acknowledges that health needs evolve over time. Whether you're diving into the initial phases for rapid results or navigating maintenance stages for long-term success, your approach is flexible and adaptive. This section explores the concept of a phased approach within the Atkins framework, allowing you to customize your journey based on current health objectives and future aspirations.

Personalized Meal Planning for Sustainable Living

Meal planning becomes a cornerstone of your toolkit, ensuring that your dietary choices align with your preferences, lifestyle, and health goals. Your toolkit guides you in crafting personalized meal plans, incorporating a variety of nutrient-dense foods, and adapting your approach to accommodate different phases, ensuring sustainability and enjoyment throughout your health adventure.

Tailoring Carbohydrate Intake to Your Lifestyle

Your lifestyle is unique, and your toolkit recognizes the importance of tailoring carbohydrate intake to fit seamlessly into your daily routines. Whether you're an active individual with specific energy needs or someone who values culinary diversity, your approach to carbohydrates is personalized, ensuring that the Atkins principles enhance, rather than disrupt, your lifestyle.

Mindset Mastery: Shaping Your Attitude for Lifelong Vitality

In the ageless vitality journey, mindset matters. Your toolkit emphasizes the power of a positive attitude, resilience in the face of challenges, and a commitment to lifelong learning. This section explores how your mindset can shape the trajectory of your health adventure, influencing your choices, habits, and overall well-being.

Your Invitation to Ageless Vitality

As you craft your personal Atkins toolkit for a lifelong health adventure, you're not just adopting a diet; you're embracing a transformative approach to well-being. This chapter concludes with an invitation to embark on your ageless vitality journey, armed with a toolkit tailored to your unique needs. By integrating strategic principles, customization, and a positive mindset, you're poised to navigate the twists and turns of life with resilience, vitality, and a commitment to ageless well-being.